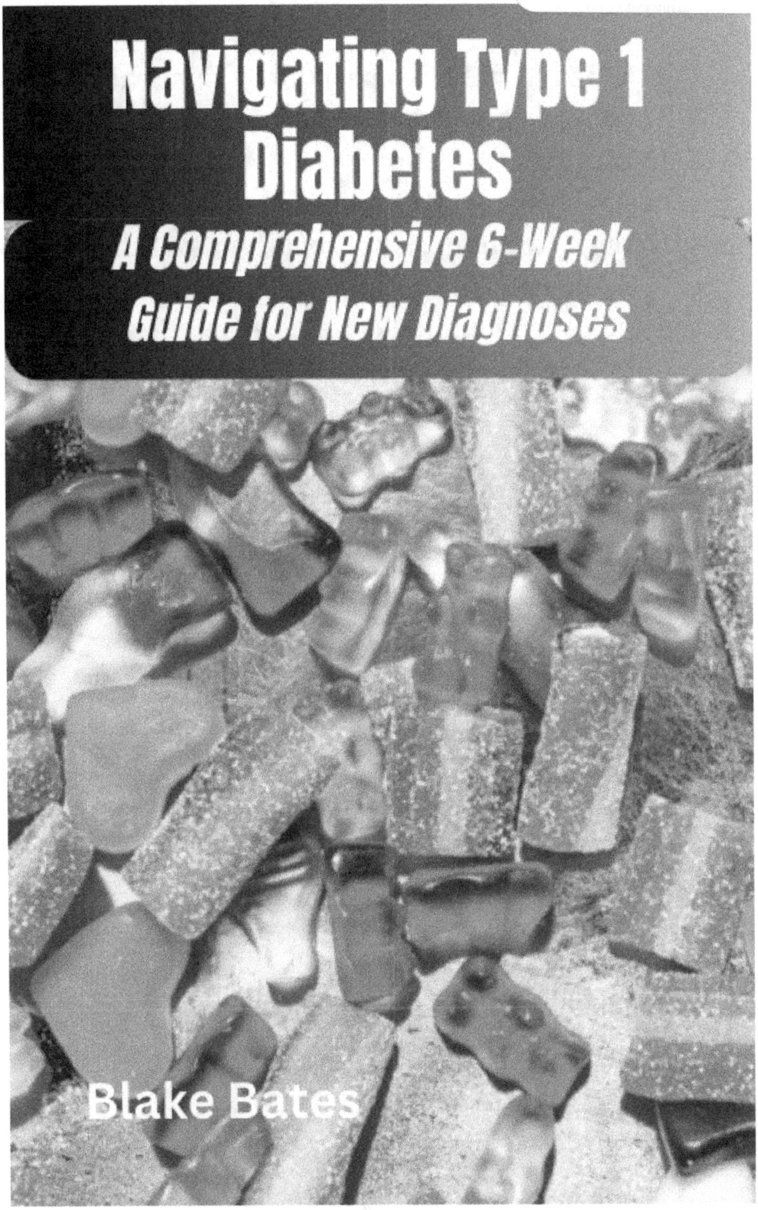

Navigating Type 1 Diabetes
A Comprehensive 6-Week Guide for New Diagnoses

Blake Bates

Copyright Page

Acknowledgements

Writing a book isn't a single travel; it's a collaborative exertion bolstered by the liberality, support, and expertise of various people. As I take a minute to precise my appreciation, I am reminded of the profound impact each individual has had on bringing this project to fruition.

To begin with and preeminent, I amplify my ardent appreciation to my family for their faithful back and understanding amid the endless hours went through inundated in investigate and composing. Your support given the establishment for this endeavor.

To my companions and colleagues who advertised profitable bits of knowledge, shared their encounters, and given helpful criticism – your commitments have improved the substance and included profundity to the story. I am monstrously thankful for your liberality.

An extraordinary thank you to the healthcare experts and specialists who benevolently shared their knowledge, ensuring the precision and unwavering quality of the data displayed. Your devotion to progressing wellbeing and well-being is genuinely commendable.

I expand my appreciation to the individuals of the diabetes community, whose stories and flexibility rouse the heart of this book. Your shared encounters serve as a guide for others exploring comparative ways.

To the publishing group whose ability changed words into an unmistakable creation – thank you for your direction, tolerance, and commitment to brilliance.

This book is dedicated to all those who endeavor for a more beneficial, more informed, and engaged life. May it serve as a source of motivation, direction, and support in your travel.

Thank you, from the depths of my heart, to everybody who played a part, huge or little, in bringing this book to life. Your affect is immense.

With appreciation,

Blake Bates

Table of Contents

Introduction

Within the embroidered artwork of human wellbeing, where each string speaks to an interesting travel, the story of those living with type 1 diabetes weaves a story of resilience, versatility, and triumph. This book may be a compass for those exploring the scene of type 1 diabetes, advertising not as it were direction on the viable perspectives of overseeing the condition but too knowledge into the passionate and mental measurements of this persistent immune system clutter.

As we set out on this investigation, it's basic to recognize the challenges confronted by people with type 1 diabetes, from the complexities of affront administration to the everyday choices around nourishment, work out, and generally well-being. In any case, within these challenges lie openings for strengthening, development, and a dynamic life.

This book may be a perfection of information, encounters, and master experiences pointed at cultivating a profound understanding of type 1 diabetes. It looks to enable people with viable procedures, all-encompassing approaches, and a different collection of diabetes-friendly formulas. Past the clinical viewpoints, it digs into the passionate texture of living with an incessant condition, recognizing the highs and lows, and giving instruments for flexibility.

Our travel together includes the taking after chapters:

Type 1 Diabetes

A foundational chapter that enlightens the immune system beginning of the condition, its common indications, and the pivotal part of affront.

• Preparing for the Travel:

Preparing perusers with the knowledge and mindset required to explore the challenges of living with type 1 diabetes.

• Culinary Investigation:

A culinary journey highlighting a curated collection of tasty formulas planned with diabetes administration in intellect.

• Grasping Alter:

Tending to the passionate scene, investigating adapting techniques, and advertising direction on developing a positive attitude.

• Feasible Wellness:

A guide for long-term well-being, centering on versatile techniques, nonstop learning, and building a steady community.

This book isn't only a direct; it's a welcome to embark on a travel of self-discovery, strengthening, and strength. It's a confirmation to the quality inside each individual confronting the complexities of type 1 diabetes. As we explore the pages ahead, may this asset serve as a companion, advertising experiences, motivation, and a guide for a satisfying life with type 1 diabetes.

Reason for the Book

This book endeavors to be a directing light for people exploring the complexities of overseeing type 1 diabetes. Through a comprehensive investigation of viable techniques, bits of knowledge from healthcare experts, and a curated collection of diabetes-friendly formulas, the essential purpose is to engage perusers with the information and devices required to take charge of their wellbeing.

1. Instruction and Understanding:

The book points to demystify the complicated scene of type 1 diabetes, giving clear and open data approximately the condition, its conclusion, and the basic standards of its administration. By cultivating a profound understanding, perusers can make educated choices around their health.

2. Strengthening Through Self-Care:

Central to the book's reason is the strengthening of people to become active members in their wellbeing travel. It offers practical advice on way of life alterations, dietary choices, and compelling self-care hones, empowering perusers to embrace a proactive part in overseeing their diabetes.

3. Holistic Well-Being:

Past the physical viewpoints of diabetes administration, the book digs into the enthusiastic and mental measurements of living with an unremitting condition. It gives devices for adapting with stretch, cultivating enthusiastic versatility, and keeping up a positive mindset—a fundamentally portion of all-encompassing well-being.

4. Culinary Investigation for Wellbeing:

With a curated collection of formulas, the book looks for to rethink the relationship between people and their dinners. It empowers a positive and pleasant approach to cooking and eating, emphasizing scrumptious, diabetes-friendly alternatives that adjust with wholesome needs.

5. Long-Term Wellness:

The extreme objective is to direct perusers towards economical hones for long-term wellness. By tending to the challenges of diabetes with versatility, flexibility, and a persistent learning attitude, people can build an establishment for a solid and satisfying life.

6. Community and Back:

Recognizing the significance of community back, the book fosters a sense of association among perusers. It recognizes the shared encounters inside the diabetes community and aims to form a supportive space for learning, sharing, and developing together.

In pith, this book aspires to be a companion, advertising not as it were down to earth advice but also motivation and support for the travel ahead. It is outlined to be a comprehensive asset that prepares individuals with the devices they ought to grasp alter, develop strength, and explore the way to long-term well-being with certainty.

Understanding Type 1 Diabetes

Type 1 diabetes could be a chronic autoimmune condition characterized by the body's immune framework assaulting and wrecking the insulin-producing beta cells within the pancreas. Affront could be a hormone fundamental for directing blood sugar (glucose) levels. When the beta cells are harmed, the body can no longer produce adequate affront, driving to lifted blood sugar levels.

Key Highlights of Type 1 Diabetes

1. Immune system Beginning:

Type 1 diabetes is fundamentally an immune system clutter, where the safe framework erroneously distinguishes and devastates the insulin-producing beta cells within the pancreas.

2. Affront Lack:

The need of affront generation comes about in a failure to direct blood sugar levels successfully.

Affront is crucial for facilitating the passage of glucose into cells, where it is utilized for vitality.

3. Onset in Childhood or Youth:

Type 1 diabetes regularly creates in childhood or adolescence, although it can happen at any age. It accounts for a critical extent of diabetes cases in children.

4. Hereditary Inclination:

There's a hereditary component to type 1 diabetes, but it isn't exclusively decided by genetics. Environmental factors, such as viral diseases, may trigger the immune system reaction in people with a hereditary inclination.

Common Indications:

1. Intemperate Thirst (Polydipsia):

People with type 1 diabetes regularly involvement expanded thirst due to the body's endeavor to kill overabundance glucose through pee.

2. Visit Urination (Polyuria):

Lifted blood sugar levels lead to expanded pee generation, causing visit trips to the lavatory.

3. Unexplained Weight Misfortune:

The body starts to break down muscle and fat for vitality when it cannot utilize glucose legitimately, coming about in weight misfortune.

4. Extraordinary Starvation (Polyphagia):

In spite of expanded nourishment utilization, the body's cells are denied of glucose, driving to diligent starvation.

5. Weariness and Shortcoming:

Inadequately glucose utilization by cells can result in weakness and shortcoming.

Administration:

1. Affront Treatment:

The foundation of type 1 diabetes administration is affront treatment. People with type 1 diabetes ought to infuse affront or utilize an affront pump to control blood sugar levels.

2. Blood Sugar Observing:

Normal checking of blood sugar levels is pivotal for altering affront measurements and keeping up ideal control.

3. Sound Way of life:

Embracing a solid way of life, counting an adjusted count calories, customary work out, and stretch administration, contributes to in general well-being and blood sugar control.

4. Persistent Learning:

Overseeing type 1 diabetes requires ceaseless learning and adjustment to changing circumstances. Remaining educated almost unused innovations and treatment alternatives is fundamental.

Understanding type 1 diabetes includes recognizing its immune system beginning, the significance of affront, and the requirement for careful administration to avoid complications. Continuous bolster from healthcare experts, a solid bolster framework, and a proactive approach to self-care contribute to a satisfying life with type 1 diabetes

Understanding the Conclusion of Diabetes

1. Introduction to Diabetes

• Diabetes may be a predominant, incessant condition characterized by hoisted blood sugar levels.

• It regularly creates without quick discernible symptoms, making early location vital.

2. Types of Diabetes

• Type 1 Diabetes:

An immune system condition where the body's resistant framework assaults and crushes insulin-producing cells.

• Type 2 Diabetes:

Related with affront resistance and lacking affront generation; regularly connected to way of life components.

• Other Types:

Gestational diabetes amid pregnancy and less common shapes like MODY.

3. Signs and Side effects

• Side effects change but may incorporate intemperate thirst, visit urination, unexplained weight misfortune, and weakness.

• Recognizing these signs is fundamental for early determination and mediation.

4. Symptomatic Tests

• Blood Glucose Tests:

Fasting, irregular, and OGTT give quick bits of knowledge into blood sugar levels.

• A1C Test:

Offers a broader picture of normal blood sugar over a few months.

5. Hazard Components and Inclination

• Hereditary Variables:

Family history can increment defenselessness.

• Way of life Impacts:

Stationary way of life, destitute dietary choices, and weight raise hazard.

6. The Part of Healthcare Suppliers

• Setting up a relationship with a healthcare group is essential.

• Normal check-ups and open communication guarantee viable administration.

7. Psychosocial effect of Determination

• Passionate reactions to diagnosis are different, extending from stun to acknowledgment.

• Building a strong bolster framework is crucial for mental and enthusiastic well-being.

8. Stages of Acknowledgment

• Acknowledgment may be a preparation that people navigate differently.

• Grasping the determination may be a pivotal step toward compelling self-management.

9. Instructive Assets for Understanding Diabetes

• Get to legitimate sources for nonstop instruction.

• Remain educated through books, sound websites, and bolster bunches.

10. Conclusion

• Understanding the determination engages people to require charge of their wellbeing.

• Deep rooted learning, coupled with a positive attitude, shapes the establishment for successful diabetes administration and a satisfying life.

What is Type 1 Diabetes?

Type 1 Diabetes could be an unremitting immune system condition characterized by the safe framework mistakenly attacking and wrecking insulin-producing beta cells within the pancreas. Affront may be a hormone pivotal for directing blood sugar (glucose) levels within the body. As these cells are harmed, the pancreas produces small to no affront, coming about in hoisted blood sugar levels.

Key Focuses Approximately Type 1 Diabetes

1. Immune system Beginning:

Not at all like Type 2 Diabetes, which is regularly related with way of life components, Type 1 Diabetes is primarily autoimmune. The safe framework, rather than ensuring the body, turns against it, driving to the annihilation of insulin-producing cells.

2. Affront Reliance:

People with Type 1 Diabetes are insulin-dependent, meaning they require outside affront to oversee their blood sugar levels. This will be conveyed through infusions or an affront pump.

3. Onset:

Type 1 Diabetes frequently shows in childhood or puberty, in spite of the fact that it can happen at any age. The precise cause remains vague, and there's no known way to anticipate the immune system assault that triggers the condition.

4. Side effects:

Common indications incorporate over the top thirst, frequent urination, unexplained weight misfortune, weariness, and expanded starvation. Incite diagnosis and administration are pivotal to anticipate complications.

5. Deep rooted Administration:

There's as of now no remedy for Type 1 Diabetes. Administration includes a lifelong commitment to affront treatment, blood sugar observing, an adjusted eat less, and normal work out.

Understanding Type 1 Diabetes includes recognizing it as a complex restorative condition that requires a comprehensive approach to day by day care. With progressions in restorative innovation and continuous inquire about, people with Type 1 Diabetes can lead active and satisfying lives, but constant self-management is paramount.

Chapter 1 (Week 1)
Initial Steps and Passionate Bolster

Introductory Steps

Exploring the Determination

Accepting a diabetes conclusion can be overpowering, but taking starting steps expeditiously can set the arrangement for viable administration. This stage includes:

1. Instruction:

Start by understanding the nuts and bolts of diabetes, counting the type analyzed, suggested lifestyle changes, and the importance of steady self-care.

2. Medical Guidance:

Build up standard communication with healthcare experts. Talk about treatment plans, pharmaceutical alternatives, and any prompt activities required for stabilization.

3. Blood Sugar Observing:

Learn how to screen blood sugar levels employing a glucose meter. Normal observing gives profitable insights into the impacts of nourishment, movement, and medication.

Making a Support System:

Building a Solid Establishment

1. Family and Friends:

Open Communication:

Share the determination with near family and companions. Open discourse cultivates understanding and makes a steady environment.

Inclusion:

Empower adored ones to take part in instructive sessions or bolster bunches to upgrade their understanding of diabetes.

2. Community and Peer Back:

Joining Bolster Bunches:

Interface with local or online diabetes back bunches. Sharing encounters with others confronting comparable challenges can give enthusiastic bolster and viable bits of knowledge.

Going to Workshops:

Go to workshops or seminars conducted by healthcare experts to extend information and pick up important tips for diabetes administration.

3. Mental Wellbeing Experts:

Counseling Administrations

Consider looking for the assistance of mental wellbeing experts, such as counselors or clinicians, to address the passionate effect of the conclusion.

Stretch Administration Procedures

Learn push administration procedures to manage with the passionate viewpoints of living with diabetes.

4. Healthcare Group Collaboration:

Customary Check-ins:

Schedule normal check-ins with healthcare suppliers to discuss challenges, alterations, and any emotional concerns.

Including a Diabetes Teacher:

Lock in with a diabetes teacher who can provide personalized direction and engage successful self-management.

5. Online Assets:

Advanced Back Stages:

Investigate legitimate online stages that offer information, forums, and assets for people exploring diabetes. These stages can give a sense of community and shared encounters.

Making a vigorous support system includes proactive steps and a willingness to embrace both individual and communal assets. By cultivating understanding, open communication, and collaboration with healthcare experts, people can set out on their diabetes travel with a solid foundation of enthusiastic and commonsense back.

Making a Bolster Framework

Family and Companions

Building a Relationship with Healthcare Suppliers

Building a solid and collaborative relationship with healthcare suppliers is paramount for compelling diabetes administration. This includes proactive engagement, clear communication, and shared understanding. Here's a direct on setting up and sustaining this crucial relationship:

1. Selecting a Diabetes Care Group:

Choose healthcare professionals with ability in diabetes care, counting endocrinologists, diabetes educators, and dietitians.

Consider variables such as experience, notoriety, and compatibility with your needs.

2. Open and Fair Communication:

Share your complete restorative history, way of life, and any concerns transparently together with your healthcare group.

Viable communication shapes the foundation for personalized and focused on diabetes care.

3. Customary Check-ups and Observing:

Go to planned arrangements as exhorted by your healthcare suppliers.

Standard check-ups allow for continuous checking of your diabetes administration arrange and the opportune alteration of strategies.

4. Effectively Taking an interest in Decision-Making:

Be a dynamic member in choices related to your diabetes management.

Collaborate along with your healthcare group to set reasonable objectives and create a personalized care plan.

5. Get it Treatment Options:

Pick up a comprehensive understanding of the accessible treatment alternatives.

Examine the aces and cons of each treatment, counting medicine, affront treatment, and lifestyle alterations.

6. Inquire Questions:

Do not hesitate to ask questions about your condition, treatment choices, and any concerns you'll have.

An educated understanding is better equipped to effectively take part in their claim care.

7. Seek Clarification on Medications:

Get it the reason, dosage, and potential side effects of endorsed medicines.

Guarantee you're comfortable with the endorsed treatment plan some time recently execution.

8. Crisis Readiness:

Examine and have a clear understanding of crisis conventions, particularly in cases of severe hypoglycemia or other diabetes-related crises.

Keep crisis contact data promptly accessible.

9. Customary Upgrades on Lifestyle Changes:

Keep your healthcare group educated approximately any noteworthy changes in your way of life, such as count calories, work out, or stretch levels.

This allows for alterations in your care plan to suit these changes.

10. Utilize Innovation for Observing:

Investigate and utilize innovation instruments for blood glucose observing, and share relevant information along with your healthcare suppliers.

Innovation can upgrade farther observing and encourage convenient mediations.

11. Be Proactive in Detailing Challenges:

Report any challenges or difficulties you encounter in adhering to your care arrange.

Fair feedback helps your healthcare group address impediments and tailor your administration approach.

12. Prioritize Mental Wellbeing:

Talk about the emotional impact of living with diabetes with your healthcare group.

Mental wellbeing is an integral portion of diabetes care, and tending to it upgrades overall well-being.

Building a solid relationship along with your healthcare provider guarantees that your diabetes administration is comprehensive, personalized, and adjusted together with your objectives. This collaborative approach improves the adequacy of your care plan and contributes to your general wellbeing and well-being.

Chapter 2 (Week 2)
Exploring Way of life Changes

Dietary Alterations for Diabetes Administration

Count calories plays an essential part in overseeing diabetes, affecting blood sugar levels and in general well-being. Making educated dietary alterations is fundamental for accomplishing ideal wellbeing. Here's a comprehensive direct on how to explore dietary changes for successful diabetes administration:

1. Get it Carbohydrate Tallying:

Learn the essentials of carbohydrate checking, as carbohydrates altogether affect blood sugar levels.

Recognize sources of complex carbohydrates that give maintained vitality without causing quick spikes in blood sugar.

2. Select Diabetes-Friendly Nourishments:

Prioritize nutrient-dense nourishments such as vegetables, incline proteins, entire grains, and solid fats.

Restrain the admissions of prepared nourishments, sugary snacks, and refreshments.

3. Parcel Control:

Hone parcel control to oversee calorie admissions and avoid indulging.

Utilize littler plates, bowls, and utensils to energize careful eating.

4. Investigate the Glycemic Record:

Familiarize yourself with the glycemic file to get it how diverse nourishments influence blood sugar levels.

Choose moo to medium glycemic record nourishments for a steadier blood sugar control.

5. Adjusted Suppers and Snacks:

Make adjusted suppers that incorporate a blend of carbohydrates, proteins, and sound fats.

Arrange nutritious snacks to anticipate extraordinary starvation and direct blood sugar all through the day.

6. Steady Supper Timing:

Set up normal feast times to advance steady blood sugar levels.

Maintain a strategic distance from skipping suppers to anticipate variances in blood sugar.

7. Sugar Substitutes and Choices:

Investigate sugar substitutes and options to sweeten nourishments and refreshments without causing quick spikes in blood sugar.

Utilize characteristic sweeteners such as stevia or minister natural product in balance.

8. Screen Liquor Admissions:

Devour liquor in balance and be careful of its effect on blood sugar levels.

Select light or direct drinking and dodge intemperate utilization.

9. Remain Hydrated:

Drink a satisfactory sum of water all through the day to remain hydrated.

Limit sugary drinks and prefer water, herbal teas, or imbued water.

10. Individualize Your Count calories Arrange:

Work with an enlisted dietitian or nutritionist to form a personalized slim down arrange based on your particular needs, inclinations, and way of life.

Consider variables such as social inclinations and nourishment intolerances when fitting your eat less.

11. Screen Blood Sugar Reactions:

Routinely screen your blood sugar levels to watch how distinctive nourishments affect your readings.

Utilize this data to refine your dietary choices and keep up ideal control.

12. Counsel with a Healthcare Proficient:

Routinely counsel along with your healthcare group to survey your eating less arrangement and make vital alterations.

Keep them educated around any challenges or changes in your dietary propensities.

By making mindful dietary alterations, people with diabetes can appreciate a well-balanced and fulfilling eat less while effectively overseeing blood sugar levels. Counseling with healthcare experts and joining these alterations into an all-encompassing diabetes administration arrange contributes to in general wellbeing and well-being.

Introduction to Carbohydrate Checking

Understanding carbohydrate tallying may be a principal expertise for people overseeing diabetes, particularly for those who utilize affront treatment. Carbohydrates specifically affect blood sugar levels, and being able to evaluate and control their admissions is crucial for accomplishing ideal glycemic control. Here's an introduction to carbohydrate checking and its centrality in diabetes administration:

1. What Are Carbohydrates?

Carbohydrates are one of the three fundamental macronutrients found in nourishment, nearby proteins and fats.

They incorporate sugars, starches, and strands and are an essential source of vitality for the body.

2. Part of Carbohydrates in Blood Sugar Control:

Carbohydrates are broken down into glucose amid digestion, leading to an increment in blood sugar levels.

Overseeing carbohydrate admissions is key to controlling post-meal blood sugar spikes.

3. Carbohydrate Tallying Essentials:

Carbohydrate tallying includes evaluating the grams of carbohydrates in nourishment.

This strategy permits people to coordinate their affront measurements to the sum of carbohydrates they plan to devour.

4. The Significance of Parcel Control:

Understanding parcel sizes is necessarily to exact carbohydrate checking.

Parcel control makes a difference keep up consistency in carbohydrate intake and insulin dosing.

5. Types of Carbohydrates:

Straightforward Carbohydrates:

Found in sugars like glucose and fructose, regularly in desserts and natural products.

Complex Carbohydrates:

Found in bland nourishments like grains, vegetables, and vegetables.

6. Glycemic File and Stack:

The glycemic record measures how rapidly a carbohydrate-containing nourishment raises blood sugar levels.

Combining the glycemic record with parcel estimate gives the glycemic stack, advertising a more comprehensive understanding.

7. Perusing Sustenance Names:

Nourishment names give profitable data on the overall grams of carbohydrates per serving.

Pay consideration to serving sizes and alter amounts appropriately.

8. Utilizing Carbohydrate Trades:

Carbohydrate trades offer a rearranged way to classify and number carbohydrates.

One trade regularly speaks to 15 grams of carbohydrates.

9. Persistent Glucose Observing (CGM) and Carbohydrate Following Apps:

CGM innovation and versatile apps can help in real-time following of carbohydrate admissions.

These apparatuses offer comfort and prompt input for superior administration.

10. Working with a Registered Dietitian:

Collaborate with an enlisted dietitian to develop a personalized carbohydrate checking arrange.

A dietitian can give direction on nourishment choices, supper arranging, and by and large dietary administration.

11. Altering for Fiber:

Fiber, whereas in fact a carbohydrate, includes a negligible effect on blood sugar.

• Subtracting dietary fiber grams from the entire carbohydrate number can give a more precise reflection of the impact on blood sugar.

12. Nonstop Learning and Adjustment:

Carbohydrate tallying isn't a one-size-fits-all approach; it requires continuous learning and adaptation.

Routinely screen blood sugar levels and alter carbohydrate admissions based on person reactions.

Acing carbohydrate checking engages individuals with diabetes to form educated dietary choices, advancing steady blood sugar levels and in general well-being. As an fundamentally portion of a comprehensive diabetes administration arrange, carbohydrate checking contributes to achieving and keeping up ideal glycemic control

Distinguishing Diabetes-Friendly Nourishments

When managing diabetes, making educated choices almost what to eat is significant for keeping up steady blood sugar levels and overall health. Here's a direct to assist identify diabetes-friendly nourishments that back adjusted sustenance and contribute to compelling diabetes administration:

1. Entire Grains:

Examples: Quinoa, brown rice, oats, and entirety wheat.

Why: Wealthy in fiber and supplements, entire grains have a more continuous effect on blood sugar levels.

2. Non-Starchy Vegetables:

Examples: Verdant greens, broccoli, cauliflower, peppers, and zucchini.

Why: Moo in carbohydrates and tall in fiber, vitamins, and minerals.

3. Incline Proteins:

Examples: Chicken, turkey, fish, tofu, and vegetables.

Why: Protein makes a difference keep up satiety and has negligible effect on blood sugar levels.

4. Sound Fats:

Examples: Avocado, nuts, seeds, and olive oil.

Why: Solid fats contribute to heart wellbeing and offer assistance stabilize blood sugar.

5. Natural products in Balance:

Examples: Berries, cherries, apples, and pears.

Why: Whereas natural products contain normal sugars, their fiber substance mitigates the effect on blood sugar.

6. Dairy or Dairy Options:

Examples: Low-fat or fat-free yogurt, drain, and cheese.

Why: Great sources of calcium and protein with direct carbohydrate substance.

7. Legumes:

Examples: Lentils, chickpeas, and dark beans.

Why: High in fiber and protein, giving a moderate release of vitality.

8. Sweet Potatoes:

Why: A nutrient-rich alternative to standard potatoes, advertising fiber and basic vitamins.

9. Angle Wealthy in Omega-3 Greasy Acids:

Examples: Salmon, mackerel, and sardines.

Why: Omega-3s back heart wellbeing and may have anti-inflammatory impacts.

10. Eggs

Why: A protein-rich nourishment that can be arranged in different ways.

11. Water

Why: Remaining hydrated is basic for by and large wellbeing and can offer assistance control craving.

12. Portion-Controlled Snacks:

Examples: Nuts, seeds, Greek yogurt, or crude vegetables with hummus.

Why: Snacks with an adjustment of protein and fiber can offer assistance keep up blood sugar levels between suppers.

13. Herbs and Flavors:

Examples: Cinnamon, turmeric, and ginger.

Why: A few spices may have potential benefits for blood sugar control.

14. Non-Caloric Refreshments:

Examples: Water, herbal teas, and dark coffee.

Why: Hydration without included sugars helps control calorie admissions.

15. Nourishments with Moo Glycemic Index:

Examples: Cherries, yogurt, and vegetables.

Why: Low-GI foods cause a slower rise in blood sugar levels.

16. Disapproving Parcel Sizes:

Why: Controlling parcel sizes makes a difference oversee calorie admissions and avoids overeating.

Recognizing diabetes-friendly nourishments includes considering their effect on blood sugar levels, dietary substance, and generally contribution to a well-balanced count calories. Standard meeting with healthcare experts and dietitians ensures personalized dietary proposals adjusted with individual wellbeing objectives and inclinations.

Work out and Movement in Diabetes Administration

Standard physical action could be a foundation of viable diabetes administration. Locks in in work out offers a heap of benefits, from making strides affront affectability to promoting overall well-being. Here's a comprehensive direct on joining work out and movement into a diabetes administration arrange:

1. Types of Work out

High-impact Work out:

Exercises that increment heart rate and breathing, such as brisk strolling, cycling, swimming, and moving.

Strength Preparing:

Resistance works out utilizing weights or body weight to construct muscle quality.

Flexibility and Adjust Works out:

Extending and balance-focused exercises to enhance adaptability and avoid wounds.

2. Setting up a Schedule:

Create a steady work out schedule, pointing for at slightest 150 minutes of moderate-intensity oxygen consuming action per week.

Incorporate quality preparing works out at slightest twice a week.

3. Individualized Approach:

Tailor work out plans to person inclinations, wellness levels, and health conditions.

Counsel with healthcare experts to guarantee security and appropriateness of chosen exercises.

4. Benefits of Work out:

Progressed Affront Affectability:

Work out makes a difference cells utilize insulin more successfully, controlling blood sugar levels.

Weight Administration:

Customary action contributes to weight control, a key figure in diabetes administration.

Cardiovascular Wellbeing:

Work out improves heart wellbeing by moving forward circulation and diminishing the chance of cardiovascular complications.

5. Observing Blood Sugar Levels:

Regularly monitor blood sugar levels, particularly some time recently and after work out.

Learn how distinctive types of exercise affect blood sugar to create informed adjustments.

6. Timing of Work out:

Consider the timing of dinners concerning work out to prevent hypoglycemia (moo blood sugar).

Post-meal walks can help in blood sugar control.

7. Hydration:

Remain well-hydrated before, amid, and after work out.

Satisfactory hydration bolsters by and large wellbeing and makes a difference direct body temperature amid physical movement.

8. Warm-Up and Cool Down:

Start each work out session with a warm-up to plan the body.

Incorporate a cool-down period to steadily lower heart rate and anticipate post-exercise hypotension.

9. Wear Suitable Footwear:

Select steady and comfortable footwear, particularly on the off chance that locks in in weight-bearing works out.

Proper shoes diminish the hazard of foot complications associated with diabetes.

10. Consolidating Way of life Action:

Incorporate way of life exercises like strolling more, taking the stairs, or planting. - These exercises contribute to daily physical action levels.

11. Discussion with Healthcare Group:

Illuminate healthcare suppliers approximately the exercise plan and look for direction on adjusting exercises to person wellbeing needs. - Normal check-ups ensure adjustments to the exercise arrange if necessary.

12. Pleasant Exercises:

Choose exercises that bring bliss and fulfillment. - Pleasant works out are more likely to become a steady portion of lifestyle.

13. Accomplice or Bunch Exercises:

Engage in work out with an accomplice or connect gather exercises. - Social back improves inspiration and makes work out more pleasant.

Consolidating exercise and activity into a diabetes management arrange may be an all-encompassing approach that contributes to improved glucose control, upgraded in general wellbeing, and expanded quality of life. Individualized and pleasant exercises make regular exercise a maintainable and advantageous portion of diabetes care.

Fitting Work out to Diabetes Administration

Adjusting work out schedules to person needs and considering the particular challenges of diabetes is fundamental for successful administration. Here's a custom fitted direct on joining work out into diabetes care:

1. Meeting with Healthcare Experts:

Sometime recently beginning any work out program, counsel with healthcare suppliers to guarantee it adjusts with person wellbeing objectives and restorative conditions.

Talk about any pre-existing complications such as neuropathy or cardiovascular issues.

2. Choosing Reasonable Exercises:

Elect exercises that suit physical wellness levels, inclinations, and any existing wellbeing concerns.

Low-impact works out like strolling, swimming, or cycling are frequently well-suited for people with diabetes.

3. Observing Blood Sugar Levels:

Routinely screen blood sugar levels, particularly some time recently and after work out.

Understanding how diverse exercises affect blood sugar permits for superior administration.

4. Adjusting High-impact and Quality Preparing:

Combine oxygen consuming works out (e.g., brisk strolling, cycling) with quality preparing to improve generally wellness.

Quality preparing moves forward muscle mass and contributes to way better blood sugar control.

5. Timing of Work out Sessions:

Consider planning work out sessions deliberately, such as after suppers or when blood sugar levels are more steady.

Adjust work out timing based on person reactions.

6. Progressive Movement:

Start with reasonable work out lengths and power, continuously expanding over time.

Dodge sudden, seriously workouts that will lead to variances in blood sugar.

7. Hydration and Nourishment:

Remain well-hydrated some time recently, amid, and after work out.

Arrange meals and snacks to adjust with work out sessions, anticipating hypoglycemia or hyperglycemia.

8. Acknowledgment of Hypoglycemia Side effects:

Be mindful of indications of hypoglycemia (moo blood sugar) amid and after work out.

Carry fast-acting glucose sources in case of crises.

9. Customary Foot Checks:

People with diabetes ought to conduct standard foot checks, particularly in case locks in in weight-bearing works out.

Legitimate footwear is significant to avoid foot complications.

10. Post-Exercise Observing:

Screen blood sugar levels post-exercise to survey the effect on glucose control. - Alter future work out plans based on person reactions.

11. Adaptability and Adjust Works out:

Incorporate adaptability and adjust works out, such as yoga or tai chi, to improve generally well-being. - These works out can be useful for people with diabetes-related complications.

12. Group Sports and Social Exercises:

Lock in in group sports or social exercises to create work out more agreeable. - Social bolster can improve inspiration and adherence to a customary workout schedule.

13. Adjustments for Age and Wellness Level:

Consider adjustments for age-related changes or wellness confinements. - Tailor works out to person capabilities, guaranteeing security and maintainability.

14. Proficient Direction:

Consider working with wellness experts or certified diabetes teachers who specialize in work out programming for people with diabetes. - Personalized direction improves the viability and security of the work out arrange.

15. Normal Reevaluation:

Frequently reassess and alter the work out arrange based on changes in wellbeing status, wellness levels, or person objectives. - Persistent adjustment guarantees long-term victory in diabetes administration through work out.

Fitting work out to diabetes administration includes a personalized and versatile approach. By considering person needs, inclinations, and wellbeing status, people can make a maintainable workout schedule that bolsters generally well-being and contributes to successful diabetes care.

Coordination Physical Action into Lifestyle for Diabetes Management

Incorporating physical movement into day by day schedules may be a down to earth and economical way to oversee diabetes. By consistently mixing work out with regular exercises, people can promote overall wellbeing and improve blood sugar control. Here's a direct on coordination physical movement into daily life for compelling diabetes administration:

1. Select Dynamic Transportation:

Prefer strolling, cycling, or utilizing open transportation for commuting.

Stop assist absent from goals to include additional steps to your day.

2. Take Brief Movement Breaks:

Set updates to stand up and move each hour, particularly on the off chance that locked in in stationary work.

Extend or take a brief walk to break up delayed periods of sitting.

3. Stairs Rather than Lifts:

Select stairs over lifts at whatever point conceivable.

Climbing stairs is a fabulous way to consolidate cardiovascular workout into every day schedules.

4. Walk Gatherings:

Conduct strolling gatherings, either outside or inside the working environment.

Combining talks with physical movement advances imagination and efficiency.

5. Dynamic Commuting:

On the off chance that doable, walk or cycle to adjacent goals rather than employing a vehicle.

This not as it were includes physical action but too decreases natural affect.

6. Family Chores as Work out:

See family chores as openings for physical activity.

Vacuuming, clearing, and cultivating are successful ways to remain dynamic.

7. Take the Long Course:

Want longer courses when walking within buildings or from one area to another.

Grasp the opportunity for additional steps.

8. Work area Works out:

Consolidate basic work area works out, such as situated leg lifts or extending, amid work hours.

These works out offer assistance combat the impacts of drawn out sitting.

9. Dynamic Hobbies:

Select side interests that include development, such as moving, planting, or playing a melodic instrument.

Leisure activities can twofold as pleasant physical exercises.

10. Family and Social Exercises:

Arrange dynamic trips with family and companions, such as hiking, biking, or playing sports. - Make social occasions centered on exercises instead of inactive occasions.

11. Utilize Commercial Breaks:

Amid tv breaks, lock in in straightforward works out like squats, lunges, or walking in place. - Turn sedentary minutes into openings for movement.

12. Walk and Conversation:

When on the phone, walk around the room or exterior. - This includes steps to your daily total without disturbing your schedule.

13. Move Sessions:

Consolidate move into every day schedules, whether it's whereas cooking, cleaning, or basically enjoying music. - Dancing could be a fun and successful way to boost physical movement.

14. Wellness Apps and Contraptions:

Utilize wellness apps or wearable contraptions to track every day steps and set movement objectives. - These apparatuses give inspiration and offer assistance screen advance.

15. Arrange Dynamic Trips:

Select recreational exercises for trips, such as climbing, biking, or exploring nature trails. - Combine relaxation with physical movement for a well-rounded encounter.

16. Careful Strolling:

Hone careful strolling, centering on each step and your environment. - This careful approach upgrades both physical and mental well-being.

By coordination physical activity into way of, life people can make work out a common and agreeable portion of their schedules. These little, reliable endeavors contribute altogether to diabetes administration, advancing by and large wellbeing and lessening the risk of complications.

Chapter 3 (Week 3)
The Part of Pharmaceutical and Affront Administration in Diabetes Care

Medicine and affront administration play a significant role in controlling blood sugar levels and anticipating complications in people with diabetes. Understanding how to effectively utilize medications and insulin is basic for a comprehensive diabetes care arrange. Here's a guide on their noteworthiness and best hones:

1. Medicine Types:

• Verbal Medicines:

Different classes, such as metformin, sulfonylureas, and DPP-4 inhibitors, offer assistance oversee blood sugar levels.

• Injectable Medicines:

GLP-1 receptor agonists and SGLT-2 inhibitors are cases of injectable solutions that can be utilized either alone or in combination with other medicines.

2. Affront Treatment:

• Basal Affront:

Gives a moderate, consistent discharge of affront to oversee fasting blood sugar levels.

• Bolus Affront:

Managed some time recently suppers to address postprandial glucose spikes.

• Combination Treatment:

A few people may require a combination of basal and bolus insulin to accomplish ideal control.

3. Individualized Medication Plans:

• Pharmaceutical plans ought to be custom-made to person needs, taking under consideration variables like age, way of life, and coexisting wellbeing conditions.

• Customary adjustments may be vital based on changes in wellbeing status and reaction to medicines.

4. Timing and Consistency:

• Reliable timing of medicine organization is vital for keeping up stable blood sugar levels.

• Take after healthcare supplier recommendations regarding when and how to require medicines.

5. Checking Blood Sugar Levels:

• Routinely screen blood sugar levels as coordinated by healthcare experts.

• Observing makes a difference assess the viability of medicines and guides adjustments.

6. Way of life and Medicine Concordance:

• Facilitate pharmaceutical plans with every day schedules, suppers, and physical action.

• Make an agreeable relationship between way of life choices and medicine administration.

7. Adherence to Endorsed Measurements:

• Adhere to endorsed dosages and enlightening for drugs.

• Lost dosages or changing pharmaceutical without counseling healthcare suppliers can disturb blood sugar control.

8. Hypoglycemia Mindfulness:

• Get it the signs and side effects of hypoglycemia (low blood sugar).

• Take prompt action with a fast-acting glucose source in case hypoglycemia happens.

9. Communication with Healthcare Suppliers:

• Keep up open communication with healthcare providers about pharmaceutical adherence, side impacts, and challenges.

• Promptly report any concerns or changes in wellbeing status.

10. Customary Medicine Survey:

Schedule regular medication reviews with healthcare suppliers to survey the progressing suitability of the endorsed regimen.

Alterations may be required based on changes in health or medicine headways.

11. Understanding Affront Conveyance Strategies:

Depending on person inclinations and needs, affront can be managed through syringes, affront pens, or affront pumps. - Select a conveyance strategy that adjusts with way of life and consolation.

12. Education on Infusion Method:

Legitimate instruction on affront infusion strategy is basic for viability and security.

Pivot infusion locales to anticipate lipodystrophy.

13. Administration of Wiped out Days:

Create an arrangement for overseeing diabetes during illness, which may include adjustments to medicine doses.

Remain hydrated and screen blood sugar levels more habitually.

14. Transitioning to Affront:

For individuals transitioning to insulin, proper education and bolster are significant.

Address fears or concerns, and guarantee a smooth move to affront treatment.

15. Grasping Innovative Advances:

Investigate innovative progressions, such as continuous glucose observing (CGM) frameworks and affront pumps. - These tools can improve exactness in medicine and affront administration.

Successful medicine and affront management form a cornerstone of diabetes care. By understanding the subtleties of distinctive solutions, following to endorsed regimens, and keeping up open communication with healthcare suppliers, people can optimize blood sugar control and relieve the hazard of complications. Normal observing, instruction, and a collaborative approach contribute to fruitful pharmaceutical and affront administration in diabetes care.

Medicine Diagram in Diabetes Administration

Successfully overseeing diabetes regularly includes the utilization of medications to control blood sugar levels and anticipate complications. Here's a diagram of common solutions utilized in diabetes care:

1. Metformin:

• Sort: Verbal Pharmaceutical (Biguanide)

• Component of Activity:

Moves forward insulin sensitivity and diminishes glucose production by the liver.

• Common Brand Names:

Glucophage, Fortamet, Glumetza

2. Sulfonylureas:

• Sort: Oral Medication

• Instrument of Activity:

Stimulates the pancreas to discharge more affront.

• Common Brand Names:

Glipizide, Glyburide, Glimpizide

3. DPP-4 Inhibitors (Dipeptidyl Peptidase-4):

• Type: Verbal Medicine

• Component of Activity:

Increases affront discharge and diminishes glucose generation.

• Common Brand Names:

Sitagliptin (Januvia), Saxagliptin (Onglyza), Linagliptin (Tradjenta)

4. GLP-1 Receptor Agonists (Incretin Mimetics):

• Sort: Injectable Medicine

• Component of Activity:

Stimulates insulin discharge, smothers glucagon emission, and moderates gastric purging.

• Common Brand Names:

Exenatide (Byetta, Bydureon), Liraglutide (Victoza, Saxenda), Dulaglutide (Trulicity)

5. SGLT-2 Inhibitors (Sodium-Glucose Cotransporter-2):

• Sort: Verbal Pharmaceutical

• Component of Activity:

Blocks glucose reabsorption within the kidneys, driving to expanded glucose excretion.

• Common Brand Names:

Canagliflozin (Invokana), Dapagliflozin (Farxiga), Empagliflozin (Jardiance)

6. Affront:

• Sort: Injectable Pharmaceutical

• Mechanism of Action:

Specifically replaces or supplements the body's affront.

• Types:

• Rapid-Acting (e.g., Affront lispro, Insulin aspart)

• Short-Acting (e.g., Normal affront)

• Intermediate-Acting (e.g., NPH affront)

• Long-Acting (e.g., Affront glargine, Affront detemir)

7. Alpha-Glucosidase Inhibitors:

• Sort: Verbal Medication

• Component of Activity:

Moderates down the digestion of carbohydrates, diminishing postprandial glucose spikes.

• Common Brand Names:

Acarbose (Precose), Miglitol (Glyset)

8. Meglitinides:

• Sort: Verbal Pharmaceutical

• Instrument of Action:

Invigorates affront discharge, especially in reaction to meals.

• Common Brand Names:

Repaglinide (Prandin), Nateglinide (Starlix)

9. Thiazolidinediones (TZDs):

• Sort: Verbal Pharmaceutical

• Instrument of Activity:

Makes strides affront affectability in muscle and fat tissue.

• Common Brand Names:

Pioglitazone (Actos), Rosiglitazone (Avandia)

10. Combination Solutions:

A few drugs combine two or more classes to supply a synergistic impact and disentangle treatment regimens.

Imperative Contemplations

• Medicines may have side impacts; people ought to be mindful of potential unfavorable responses.

• Adherence to endorsed doses and plans is vital for ideal adequacy.

• Normal checking of blood sugar levels makes a difference evaluate the effect of medicines and direct alterations.

• Way of life alterations, counting slim down and work out, complement pharmaceutical treatment for comprehensive diabetes administration.

Note: Medicines and their accessibility may change by locale, and particular drugs ought to be endorsed by healthcare experts based on person wellbeing needs and contemplations. Continuously counsel with healthcare suppliers for personalized counsel and administration plans.

Introduction to Affront

Introduction to Affront in Diabetes Administration

Affront could be a hormone crucial for directing blood sugar levels within the body. In people with diabetes, the common generation or adequacy of affront is disabled, requiring the utilization of manufactured affront to oversee the condition viably. Here's an introduction to the part of affront and its significance in diabetes care:

1. Part of Affront:

• Affront is delivered by the pancreas and plays an urgent part in glucose digestion system.

• It encourages the take-up of glucose by cells, permitting them to utilize it for vitality.

• Affront moreover represses the liver from discharging intemperate glucose into the circulation system.

2. Types of Affront:

• Rapid-Acting Affront:

Starts working inside 15 minutes, crests in almost an hour, and keeps going for 2 to 4 hours.

• Short-Acting (Normal) Affront:

Begins working inside 30 minutes, crests in 2 to 3 hours, and includes a term of 3 to 6 hours.

• Intermediate-Acting Affront:

Onset is 2 to 4 hours, crest is 4 to 12 hours, and it endures around 12 to 18 hours.

• Long-Acting Affront:

Takes several hours to begin working and gives a slow, steady discharge over a more expanded period, ordinarily 24 hours.

3. Organization Strategies:

• Subcutaneous Infusions:

Most commonly managed fair beneath the skin utilizing affront syringes, pens, or pumps.

• Breathed in Affront:

A more current strategy includes breathing in affront powder through the mouth.

• Affront Pumps:

Little gadgets worn remotely that ceaselessly provide affront through a catheter set beneath the skin.

4. Signs for Affront Utilize:

• People with Type 1 diabetes, where the pancreas produces small to no affront.

• A few individuals with Type 2 diabetes may moreover require affront when verbal medicines or other injectable solutions are inadequately to control blood sugar.

5. Affront and Blood Sugar Control:

• Affront is pivotal for keeping up steady blood sugar levels.

• Appropriate insulin management makes a difference avoid hyperglycemia (tall blood sugar) and hypoglycemia (moo blood sugar).

6. Individualized Affront Plans:

• Affront regimens are exceedingly individualized, taking under consideration components like way of life, eating designs, and in general wellbeing.

• Combination therapies with different types of affront may be prescribed.

7. Challenges and Contemplations:

• Hypoglycemia Chance:

Affront, in the event that not dosed or coordinated accurately, can lead to moo blood sugar levels.

• Infusion Location Revolution:

Routinely changing infusion destinations makes a difference anticipate lipodystrophy (fat stores) and guarantees steady assimilation.

8. Progresses in Affront Innovation:

• Persistent Glucose Observing (CGM):

Combined with affront pumps, CGM permits for real-time observing and alteration of affront conveyance.

• Ultra-Rapid Affront:

More up to date details point for indeed speedier onset and shorter length, mirroring more closely the body's normal affront reaction.

In summary, Affront may be a life-saving medicine for people with diabetes, permitting them to oversee their condition effectively. Its significance lies in its capacity to imitate the normal activities of affront, making a difference control blood sugar levels and anticipating complications associated with uncontrolled diabetes. Continuously counsel with healthcare experts to decide the foremost appropriate affront regimen based on person health needs and contemplations.

Other Drugs for Type 1 Diabetes

As of my final information update in January 2022, affront remains the essential and fundamental treatment for Type 1 diabetes. People with Type 1 diabetes require affront treatment to supplant the hormone their bodies are incapable to create. In any case, inquire about and therapeutic headways proceed, and it's basic to remain educated around the most recent improvements.

Separated from affront, there can be steady drugs or developing treatments in clinical trials. These may incorporate medicines to address particular complications or innovations like closed-loop frameworks, moreover known as fake pancreas frameworks, which combine affront pumps with persistent glucose checking.

It's significant to note that any unused solutions or medications ought to be endorsed and observed by healthcare experts. On the off chance that you're seeking out for the latest information, I prescribe checking trustworthy therapeutic sources, counseling with healthcare suppliers, or alluding to later therapeutic writing for overhauls on Type 1 Diabetes medications.

Continuously consult with healthcare experts for personalized exhortation and the foremost current data custom fitted to your particular wellbeing condition and needs.

Understanding Insulin Types and Conveyance Strategies in Diabetes Management

Affront could be a basic hormone for overseeing blood sugar levels, and people with diabetes may utilize different types of insulin and conveyance strategies to attain ideal control. Here's a diagram of affront types and common conveyance strategies:

1. Types of Insulin:

• Rapid-Acting Affront:

• Cases: Affront lispro, affront aspart, affront glulisine.

• Onset: 15 minutes.

• Crest: 1-2 hours.

• Length: 2-4 hours.

• Organization: Some time recently dinners to oversee postprandial spikes.

• Short-Acting (Normal) Affront:

• Examples: Normal affront.

• Onset: 30 minutes.

• Crest: 2-3 hours.

• Length: 3-6 hours.

• Organization: Sometime recently dinners to cover glucose from food intake.

• Intermediate-Acting Affront:

• Cases: NPH (Unbiased Protamine Hagedorn) affront.

• Onset: 2-4 hours.

• Top: 4-12 hours.

• Length: 12-18 hours.

• Organization: Frequently utilized as a basal affront, providing coverage between dinners and overnight.

• Long-Acting Affront:

• Cases: Affront glargine, insulin detemir, insulin degludec.

• Onset: Changes (some have a progressive onset over hours).

• Top: Negligible crest or no peak.

• Duration: Up to 24 hours.

• Organization: Used for basal affront needs, giving a consistent discharge all through the day.

• Ultra-Rapid Affront:

• Examples: Affront lispro-aabc (Lyumjev).

• Onset: Indeed faster than conventional rapid-acting insulins.

• Top: Quick.

• Term: Brief.

• Organization: Sometime recently suppers for fast and short-lived activity.

2. Affront Conveyance Strategies:

• Subcutaneous Infusions:

• Method: Managed fair beneath the skin utilizing affront syringes, insulin pens, or affront pumps.

• Recurrence: Different infusions all through the day for those on different every day infusions (MDI) or continuous infusion for pump clients.

• Affront Pens:

• Depiction: Expendable or reusable pen-shaped gadgets that contain pre-loaded insulin cartridges.

• Advantages: Helpful, tactful, and simple to utilize.

• Affront Pumps:

• Description: Little gadgets worn remotely that persistently deliver insulin through a catheter put beneath the skin.

• Points of interest: Mirrors the function of a healthy pancreas by giving a consistent basal rate and permitting for precise bolus dosages.

• Breathed in Affront:

• Strategy: Affront conveyed through inward breath utilizing an inhaler gadget.

• Points of interest: Non-invasive, an elective for those who lean toward not to infuse.

3. Variables Affecting Affront Choice:

• Way of life Components: Every day schedule, feast designs, and movement levels.

• Person Needs: The interesting affront necessities of each individual.

• Treatment Objectives: Whether focusing on tight glucose control or more adaptable administration.

• Healthcare Supplier Proposals: Guidance from healthcare experts based on person wellbeing conditions.

Understanding the distinctive affront types and conveyance strategies is significant for individuals with diabetes and their healthcare providers to make personalized treatment plans that best fit their needs and lifestyles. Standard communication with healthcare experts guarantees alterations can be made as required to attain ideal blood sugar control.

Creating a Personalized Affront Schedule

Planning a personalized affront schedule is a collaborative process involving people with diabetes and their healthcare suppliers. Fitting the affront regimen to individual needs, way of life, and wellbeing status is fundamental for accomplishing ideal blood sugar control. Here's a direct on making a personalized affront schedule:

1. Comprehensive Evaluation:

• Conduct an intensive evaluation of the individual's wellbeing, counting generally physical wellbeing, way of life, eating propensities, and day by day schedules.

• Consider components such as age, occupation, work out propensities, and any coexisting therapeutic conditions.

2. Type of Diabetes:

• Decide whether the person has Type 1 or Type 2 diabetes, as affront needs and administration procedures may contrast.

3. Insulin Types and Combinations:

• Collaborate with healthcare suppliers to select the most fitting types of affront.

• Consider a combination of rapid-acting, short-acting, intermediate-acting, and/or long-acting affront based on person requirements.

4. Basal-Bolus Approach:

Implement a basal-bolus affront approach, which includes:

• Basal Affront: Giving a steady background affront level.

• Bolus Affront: Addressing mealtime glucose spikes.

5. Timing of Affront Injections:

• Build up a reliable plan for insulin administration.

• Adjust affront dosages with dinners and snacks to preserve steady blood sugar levels all through the day.

6. Individualized Dosing:

• Decide person affront affectability and carbohydrate-to-insulin proportions.

• Alter affront measurements based on components like physical action, push, ailment, and changes in schedule.

7. Flexibility and Versatility:

• Design a schedule that gives adaptability to oblige varieties in standard of living.

• Permit for alterations in affront measurements when required, beneath the direction of healthcare suppliers.

8. Mealtime Affront:

• Regulate rapid-acting or short-acting affront some time recently suppers to address postprandial glucose spikes.

• Consider insulin-to-carbohydrate proportions to decide fitting dosages.

9. Bedtime or Overnight Affront:

• Incorporate long-acting or intermediate-acting affront to preserve steady blood sugar levels overnight.

• Alter sleep time insulin doses based on nighttime blood sugar designs.

10. Observing and Standard Audits:

Frequently monitor blood sugar levels using self-monitoring or ceaseless glucose monitoring (CGM).

Plan standard surveys with healthcare suppliers to assess the adequacy of the affront regimen.

11. Education and Strengthening:

Teach people around their affront regimen, including legitimate injection techniques, location revolution, and recognizing signs of hypo- or hyperglycemia.

Enable people to actively take part in their diabetes administration.

12. Innovation Integration:

Investigate the integration of innovation, such as affront pumps or closed-loop frameworks, based on person inclinations and needs.

13. Way of life Considerations:

Consider the effect of lifestyle factors, such as travel, work plan, and social exercises, when planning the affront schedule. - Create methodologies for overseeing affront amid extraordinary circumstances.

14. Mental and Enthusiastic Back:

Recognize the enthusiastic and mental angles of living with diabetes.

Give assets and support for adapting with the everyday challenges of affront administration.

15. Regular Communication:

Keep up open and standard communication with healthcare providers.

Instantly report any challenges, concerns, or changes in health status that will affect the affront schedule.

Making a personalized affront schedule is a continuous process that requires collaboration, flexibility, and a proactive approach to diabetes administration. By fitting the affront regimen to individual needs and cultivating a strong organization between people and healthcare suppliers, ideal blood sugar control and by and large well-being can be achieved. Continuously consult with healthcare experts for personalized advice based on person wellbeing contemplations.

Chapter 4 (Week 4)
Observing Blood Sugar Levels

The Significance of Blood Sugar Observing in Diabetes Administration

Checking blood sugar levels could be a significant perspective of overseeing diabetes successfully. Normal and precise blood sugar observing gives profitable experiences into how well an individual's diabetes treatment arrange is working and makes a difference avoid complications. Here are key reasons highlighting the significance of blood sugar observing:

Customizing Treatment Plans

• Blood sugar observing permits healthcare suppliers to tailor treatment plans to person needs.

• Alterations in medicine doses, affront regimens, or way of life adjustments can be made based on real-time glucose information.

2. Early Discovery of Hyperglycemia:

• Customary observing makes a difference recognize and address tall blood sugar levels expeditiously.

• Early mediation avoids the movement of hyperglycemia, diminishing the chance of complications such as cardiovascular issues, kidney issues, and nerve harm.

3. Anticipation of Hypoglycemia:

• Checking blood sugar levels makes a difference avoid scenes of hypoglycemia (moo blood sugar).

• Maintaining a strategic distance from unreasonably moo blood sugar is vital to avoid prompt wellbeing dangers and improve in general well-being.

4. Assessment of Mealtime Administration:

• Blood sugar readings some time recently and after dinners give bits of knowledge into the effect of dietary choices on glucose levels.

• Alterations to meal plans or affront measurements can be made based on this data.

5. Understanding Blood Sugar Designs:

• Persistent glucose checking (CGM) offers a comprehensive set of blood sugar designs all through the day and night.

• Recognizing patterns makes a difference in arranging more successful affront regimens and way of life alterations.

6. Direction for Physical Movement:

• Checking blood sugar levels some time recently, amid, and after work out makes a difference tailor physical movement plans.

• Alterations to affront measurements or carbohydrate admissions can be made to preserve steady glucose levels amid work out.

7. Bolster for Pharmaceutical Administration:

• Blood sugar observing helps in evaluating the viability of verbal medicines or affront treatment.

• Ensures individuals are utilizing the proper measurement and makes a difference avoid unfavorable impacts.

8. Individual Strengthening:

• Standard observing enables people with diabetes to effectively take part in their possess care.

• Makes a difference people get it the effect of their way of life choices on blood sugar levels.

9. Avoidance of Long-Term Complications:

• Steady blood sugar control, encouraged by observing, is vital in anticipating long-term complications such as retinopathy, nephropathy, and neuropathy.

10. Progressed Quality of Life:

Ideal blood sugar administration contributes to a moved forward quality of life.

Decreases the burden of diabetes-related side effects and minimizes the hazard of intense and constant complications.

11. Objective Setting and Accomplishment:

Checking blood sugar levels makes a difference people set reasonable glycemic targets.

Accomplishing and keeping up these targets is basic for generally wellbeing and well-being.

12. Improved Communication with Healthcare Suppliers:

Customary checking encourages significant dialogs between people with diabetes and healthcare providers.

Permits for collaborative decision-making and alterations to treatment plans.

13. Distinguishing proof of Designs and Patterns:

Following blood sugar levels over time makes a difference recognize designs and patterns, helping within the distinguishing proof of components affecting glucose control.

14. Progressed Mental Wellbeing:

Knowing and overseeing blood sugar levels successfully can emphatically affect mental wellbeing, diminishing push and uneasiness related with diabetes administration.

15. Crisis Readiness:

Blood sugar checking gives people with diabetes the capacity to identify and react to crisis circumstances, such as extreme hypoglycemia or hyperglycemia.

Therefore, customary blood sugar checking could be a foundation of viable diabetes administration. It engages people, guides treatment choices, and essentially contributes to accomplishing and keeping up ideal blood sugar control. Always counsel with healthcare suppliers to set up a fitting observing routine tailored to person needs and wellbeing considerations.

Choosing and Employing a Glucose Meter

Selecting and utilizing a glucose meter could be a vital angle of overseeing diabetes. These gadgets empower people to screen their blood sugar levels at domestic, giving important insights for successful diabetes management. Here's a comprehensive direct on choosing and employing a glucose meter:

1. Choosing a Glucose Meter:

• Exactness:

Select a meter with tall exactness. Most modern glucose meters meet exacting precision guidelines, but it's fundamental to select one that has been approved through clinical thinks about.

• Ease of Utilize:

Choose a meter that's user-friendly, with clear enlightening and clear route. Expansive, easy-to-read shows are useful.

• Test Measure:

Consider the specified blood test estimate. Meters with littler test estimate prerequisites may be preferable for those who discover blood testing challenging.

• Speed of Comes about:

Select a meter that gives speedy and dependable comes about. Quicker readings can be especially helpful for busy ways of life.

• Memory and Information Capacity:

Meters with memory capacities and information capacity capabilities allow clients to track and audit their blood sugar patterns over time.

• Estimate and Compactness:

Select a meter that suits your way of life. Compact, portable meters are helpful for on-the-go observing.

• Compatibility with Nonstop Glucose Observing (CGM):

For those utilizing CGM frameworks, consider meters that coordinated consistently with CGM information for a more comprehensive view of glucose levels.

• Taken a toll and Protections Scope:

Evaluate the fetched of the meter and associated supplies. Check on the off chance that the meter and its consumables are secured by your protections arrange.

2. Steps for Legitimate Blood Glucose Observing:

• Wash Hands:

Clean your hands thoroughly with cleanser and water. Maintain a strategic distance from utilizing alcohol-based wipes some time recently testing, as they can influence readings.

• Get ready the Spearing Gadget:

Load a lancet into the spearing gadget. Alter the profundity setting based on your skin type and the specific device instructions.

• Get ready the Test Strip:

Embed a new test strip into the meter agreeing to the manufacturer's instruction.

• Prick the Finger:

Use the spearing gadget to get a little blood test. Take after the particular enlightening for getting an adequate sample.

• Apply Blood to Test Strip:

Touch the blood drop to the assigned zone on the test strip. Guarantee the meter registers the sample.

• Hold up for Comes about:

The meter will show your blood sugar level after a brief handling time. Record the result on the off chance that required.

• Arrange of Lancet and Test Strip Properly:

Securely dispose of utilized lancets and test strips concurring to nearby directions and producer recommendations.

3. Maintenance and Investigating:

• Calibration:

A few meters require periodic calibration with control arrangements. Take after the manufacturer's instruction for calibration in case essential.

• Battery Substitution:

Screen the battery life of your glucose meter and supplant batteries instantly to guarantee exact readings.

• Cleaning:

Clean the meter and its components routinely taking after the manufacturer's rules. Dodge utilizing cruel chemicals that may damage the device.

• Quality Control:

Intermittently check the meter's precision by comparing comes about with those gotten in a healthcare setting.

• Tending to Blunder Messages:

Familiarize yourself with common blunder messages and troubleshoot issues agreeing to the meter's instruction.

4. Customary Observing and Record-Keeping:

• Recurrence of Testing:

Take after your healthcare provider's suggestions for the recurrence of blood sugar testing. This may change based on your treatment plan and person needs.

• Record Comes about:

Keep a log or utilize the meter's memory work to record blood sugar comes about. This data is important for both you and your healthcare team.

• Audit Patterns:

Occasionally audit your blood sugar patterns to recognize patterns and make informed decisions around alterations to your treatment arrange.

Choosing the correct glucose meter and utilizing it viably are imperative components of effective diabetes administration. Normal blood sugar observing enables individuals to make educated choices almost way of life, medicine, and by and large wellbeing. Continuously counsel together with your healthcare supplier for personalized direction on blood sugar checking and administration.

Understanding Blood Sugar Targets in Diabetes Administration

Blood sugar targets, frequently alluded to as glycemic targets, are particular ranges of blood glucose levels that people with diabetes point to realize and keep up. These targets play a vital part in overseeing diabetes viably and preventing complications related with fluctuating blood sugar levels. Here's a comprehensive direct to understanding blood sugar targets:

1. Individualized Targets:

• Blood sugar targets are exceedingly individualized and depend on different variables, counting the type of diabetes, age, overall wellbeing, and the nearness of any complications.

• Healthcare suppliers work collaboratively with people with diabetes to set up personalized glycemic objectives.

2. Type of Diabetes:

• Type 1 Diabetes:

For people with Type 1 diabetes, the objective is to accomplish blood sugar levels as near to the ordinary extend as conceivable. This makes a difference anticipate acute complications like hypoglycemia and long-term complications.

• Type 2 Diabetes:

Targets for people with Type 2 diabetes are for the most part more adaptable and may include an adjustment between accomplishing optimal control and minimizing the chance of hypoglycemia.

3. Ordinary Blood Sugar Extend:

• The ordinary blood sugar extend for people without diabetes typically falls between 70 and 140 mg/dL (3.9 to 7.8 mmol/L) all through the day.

• Fasting blood sugar levels (before dinners) are frequently suggested to be underneath 100 mg/dL (5.6 mmol/L).

4. A1c Objectives:

• The A1c test gives an normal of blood sugar levels over the past 2-3 months.

• A common target for A1c is underneath 7% for numerous people, but individualized objectives may shift.

5. Time-of-Day Targets:

• Targets for blood sugar levels can shift all through the day:

• Fasting (Some time recently Suppers):

Typically, the objective is to keep fasting blood sugar levels between 80 and 130 mg/dL (4.4 to 7.2 mmol/L).

• Postprandial (After Suppers):

Aim for levels below 180 mg/dL (10 mmol/L) almost 1-2 hours after beginning a meal.

6. Hypoglycemia and Hyperglycemia:

• Hypoglycemia (Moo Blood Sugar):

Maintaining a strategic distance from blood sugar levels underneath 70 mg/dL (3.9 mmol/L) makes a difference prevent symptoms of hypoglycemia, such as discombobulation and confusion.

• Hyperglycemia (Tall Blood Sugar):

Consistently tall blood sugar levels can contribute to long-term complications. Overseeing postprandial levels is especially important.

7. Adjustments for Extraordinary Circumstances:

• Targets may be balanced based on person circumstances, such as age, coexisting health conditions, and way of life variables.

• Uncommon consideration is given amid pregnancy (gestational diabetes) or when overseeing diabetes in more seasoned grown-ups.

8. Persistent Glucose Monitoring (CGM):

• CGM frameworks provide real-time data on blood sugar levels.

• They offer assistance people and healthcare suppliers make quick alterations to insulin doses or other perspectives of the treatment arrange.

9. Significance of Normal Checking:

• Standard observing of blood sugar levels at home is pivotal for accomplishing and keeping up glycemic targets.

• It permits people to create educated choices almost diet, physical action, and medication alterations.

10. Collaborative Approach:

Achieving blood sugar targets may be a collaborative exertion between people with diabetes and their healthcare providers. - Customary communication and alterations to the treatment arrange based on checking comes about are key components of fruitful diabetes administration.

11. Way of life Variables:

Healthy lifestyle choices, counting an adjusted count calories, regular physical movement, and push administration, contribute to accomplishing and keeping up blood sugar targets.

12. Regular Follow-Up:

Regular follow-up arrangements with healthcare suppliers are basic to evaluate advance, make alterations to the treatment arrange, and address any concerns.

Understanding and accomplishing blood sugar targets are indispensably to viable diabetes administration. Individualized objectives, customary checking, and a collaborative approach with healthcare providers empower people to preserve ideal blood sugar control and minimize the chance of complications related with diabetes. Always counsel along with your healthcare group to build up personalized blood sugar targets based on your one of a kind wellbeing contemplations.

Record Keeping

Viable Record Keeping in Diabetes Administration

Record keeping may be an imperative viewpoint of diabetes administration, giving important experiences into blood sugar designs, way of life variables, and the in general adequacy of the treatment arrange. Here's a comprehensive direct to compelling record keeping for people with diabetes:

1. Blood Sugar Logs:

• Keep up a day by day blood sugar log to track glucose levels at diverse times of the day.

• Record fasting, pre-meal, and postprandial (after dinners) blood sugar readings.

• Note any abnormal circumstances or components which will have affected the readings, such as stretch, sickness, or changes in medicine.

2. Feast and Nibble Records:

• Report dietary choices and parcel sizes for each dinner and nibble.

• Incorporate data around carbohydrates expended, as they altogether affect blood sugar levels.

• Note any enthusiastic or outside components impacting eating propensities.

3. Medicine and Affront Records:

• Keep a nitty gritty record of all drugs, counting dosages and timing.

• For people utilizing affront, report the type of affront, measurement, and infusion locales.

• Record any alterations made to medicine regimens based on healthcare supplier proposals.

4. Physical Action and Exercise Logs:

• Track the sort, term, and concentrated of physical exercises.

• Note the time of day when work out happens and any alterations made to affront or pharmaceutical dosages to suit physical movement.

• Record how work out impacts blood sugar levels.

5. Side effect and Feeling Logs:

• Keep a log of any indications experienced, such as signs of hypoglycemia (moo blood sugar) or hyperglycemia (tall blood sugar).

• Note sentiments of weakness, stretch, or emotional well-being, as these variables can impact blood sugar levels.

6. Normal Observing of A1c:

• Plan standard A1c tests as suggested by healthcare suppliers.

• Record A1c comes about over time to track long-term blood sugar control patterns.

7. Weight and Blood Weight Records:

• Screen weight and blood weight routinely.

• Changes in weight and blood weight can affect diabetes administration and by and large wellbeing.

8. Integration of Innovation:

• Utilize diabetes administration apps or gadgets that adjust with glucose meters or persistent glucose checking (CGM) frameworks.

• These apparatuses can consequently log and analyze information, giving a comprehensive set of diabetes management.

9. Survey and Examination:

• Frequently survey and analyze recorded information to distinguish designs, patterns, and potential zones for advancement.

• Share this data with healthcare suppliers amid check-ups for collaborative decision-making.

10. Objective Setting and Celebrating Accomplishments:

Set up short-term and long-term objectives for blood sugar control, way of life changes, and by and large well-being. - Celebrate accomplishments, no matter how little, to preserve inspiration and a positive viewpoint.

11. Communication with Healthcare Suppliers:

Share record-keeping logs with healthcare suppliers amid arrangements. - Open communication permits for alterations to treatment plans based on recorded information.

12. Crisis Readiness:

Keep a record of crisis contacts, healthcare supplier data, and an activity arrange for overseeing extraordinary blood sugar levels. - Guarantee family individuals or near contacts are mindful of crisis conventions.

13. Customary Follow-Up:

Plan normal follow-up arrangements with healthcare suppliers to examine record-keeping information and make any essential alterations to the treatment arrange.

14. Consistency and Commitment:

Steady and committed record keeping is key to inferring important experiences and optimizing diabetes administration. - Build up a schedule for logging information and adhere to it reliably.

Successful record keeping could be an effective apparatus in diabetes administration, giving an all-encompassing see of an individual's wellbeing. By keeping up nitty gritty logs and collaborating with healthcare suppliers, people with diabetes can make educated choices, track advance, and work towards accomplishing and keeping up ideal blood sugar control. Continuously counsel with healthcare experts for personalized guidance based on your special wellbeing contemplations.

Keeping a Diabetes Diary

A diabetes diary may be a capable instrument that permits people to track and oversee different perspectives of their diabetes care. By recording key data frequently, people can pick up profitable bits of knowledge, recognize designs, and make educated choices to optimize blood sugar control and generally well-being. Here's a comprehensive direct to keeping a diabetes diary:

1. Select a Journal Format:

• Select a physical diary, an advanced app, or an internet stage based on individual inclinations.

• Guarantee the chosen arrange is user-friendly and effortlessly available.

2. Incorporate Fundamental Data:

• Blood Sugar Readings:

Record blood sugar levels at diverse times of the day, counting fasting, pre-meal, and postprandial readings.

• Meal Details:

Report points of interest of dinners and snacks, counting parcel sizes, types of carbohydrates, and any deviations from the standard eat less.

• Pharmaceutical and Affront:

Note subtle elements approximately solutions, counting measurements and timings. For affront clients, record types of affront, measurement alterations, and infusion destinations.

3. Track Physical Movement:

• Record the type, term, and escalated of physical exercises.

• Incorporate any alterations made to affront or pharmaceutical dosages in reaction to work out.

4. Monitor Indications and Sentiments:

• Keep track of any indications experienced, such as signs of hypoglycemia (moo blood sugar) or hyperglycemia (tall blood sugar).

• Note sentiments of push, weariness, or passionate well-being, as these variables can impact blood sugar levels.

5. Log Dinner Timing:

• Archive the timing of suppers and snacks to identify potential relationships with blood sugar vacillations.

• Record any changes in dinner timing due to way of life components.

6. Record Hydration:

• Incorporate data around liquid admissions, particularly in case expending refreshments with included sugars or caffeine.

• Remaining enough hydrated is fundamental for generally wellbeing and can impact blood sugar direction.

7. Record Way of life Components:

• Note any critical way of life variables, such as rest designs, push levels, and changes in day by day schedules.

• Distinguish how these variables may impact blood sugar control.

8. Utilize Images or Codes:

• Create a framework of images or codes to rapidly speak to particular occasions or conditions.

• For illustration, utilize an exclamation stamp for days with tall stretch levels or a heart symbol for days with positive feelings.

9. Survey Patterns and Designs:

• Routinely audit diary sections to distinguish patterns and designs in blood sugar levels.

• Search for relationships between particular exercises, dinners, or occasions and their effect on glucose control.

10. Set Individual Objectives:

- Establish short-term and long-term objectives for blood sugar control, lifestyle changes, and generally well-being. - Utilize the diary to track advance towards these objectives.

11. Share with Healthcare Suppliers:

- Bring the diabetes diary to healthcare arrangements to share data with suppliers. - Examine designs, challenges, and successes to collaborate on refining the treatment arrange.

12. Celebrate Achievements:

Recognize and celebrate accomplishments, no matter how little. - Positive fortification contributes to inspiration and a proactive approach to diabetes administration.

13. Crisis Data:

Incorporate crisis contact data, healthcare supplier points of interest, and an activity arrange for extraordinary blood sugar levels. - Guarantee that family individuals or near contacts are mindful of this information.

14. Standard Follow-Up:

Plan standard surveys of the journal to survey advance and make any vital alterations to the treatment plan. - Consider overhauling objectives based on changing circumstances.

15. Keep up Consistency:

Consistency in journaling is vital for determining important experiences. - Set up a schedule for recording information, and commit to it reliably.

Keeping a diabetes diary could be a proactive and engaging approach to self-management. It permits individuals to effectively take an interest in their care, get it their unique diabetes designs, and make educated choices for ideal blood sugar control.

Continuously counsel with healthcare experts for personalized direction based on your interesting wellbeing contemplations.

A Present day Approach to Self-Management

In the era of progressed innovation, different advanced instruments and applications have risen to facilitate the following and administration of diabetes. Leveraging these mechanical arrangements can upgrade the exactness, effectiveness, and comfort of observing key angles of diabetes care. Here's a direct on utilizing innovation for following diabetes:

1. Glucose Checking Apps:

• Utilize glucose observing apps that adjust with glucose meters or persistent glucose checking (CGM) systems.

• These apps permit real-time following of blood sugar levels, provide trend investigations, and offer experiences into designs.

2. Diabetes Management Platforms:

• Investigate comprehensive diabetes administration stages that centralize information from different sources, counting blood sugar readings, supper logs, and physical action.

• Stages frequently offer customizable dashboards for an all-encompassing see of diabetes measurements.

3. Persistent Glucose Monitoring (CGM) Frameworks:

• Contribute in CGM frameworks that give ceaseless, real-time glucose observing.

• CGM gadgets transmit information to congruous smartphones or receivers, offering bits of knowledge into glucose patterns and potential cautions for tall or moo levels.

4. Shrewd Affront Pens:

• Consider utilizing keen affront pens that naturally record affront measurements and transmit the information to comparing smartphone apps.

• These pens streamline the tracking of affront organization and measurement alterations.

5. Portable Apps for Nourishment Following:

• Utilize portable apps particularly outlined for sustenance following to screen nourishment admissions, calculate carbohydrates, and log suppers.

• Apps can give wholesome data and offer assistance people make educated dietary choices.

6. Wellness Trackers and Wearables:

• Wear wellness trackers or smart watches to screen physical action and work out.

• These gadgets can adjust with wellbeing apps to provide a comprehensive outline of every day movement levels.

7. Medicine Update Apps:

• Set up medicine update apps to get notices for affront measurements or other medications.

• These apps can offer assistance guarantee convenient organization and adherence to endorsed pharmaceutical regimens.

8. Telehealth and Virtual Discussions:

• Lock in in telehealth or virtual meetings with healthcare suppliers for inaccessible observing and guidance.

• Virtual arrangements permit for the dialog of following information and alterations to the treatment arrange.

9. Online Diabetes Communities:

• Connect online diabetes communities or gatherings where people share their experiences and insights.

• These stages can give passionate back, down to earth tips, and recommendations for compelling following apparatuses.

10. Personalized Wellbeing Stages:

- Investigate personalized wellbeing stages that coordinated information from different sources, such as wellness, nourishment, and glucose checking. - These stages may offer progressed analytics and prescient bits of knowledge.

11. Shrewd Scales and Biometric Gadgets:

Utilize shrewd scales and biometric gadgets that sync with following apps to screen weight, blood weight, and other pertinent wellbeing metrics. - These gadgets contribute to a more comprehensive understanding of overall health.

12. Manufactured Insights (AI) Arrangements:

Investigate AI-powered arrangements that analyze following information to supply personalized suggestions. - AI calculations can distinguish designs and suggest alterations to optimize diabetes administration.

13. Information Security and Privacy Considerations:

Prioritize stages and apps with strong security measures to ensure delicate wellbeing information. - Ensure compliance with security directions and survey terms of use.

14. Standard Overhauls and Updates:

Keep following apps, gadgets, and stages up to date with the most recent computer program adaptations. - Normal overhauls regularly incorporate upgrades, bug fixes, and unused highlights.

15. Collaborate with Healthcare Suppliers:

Share followed information with healthcare suppliers during appointments. - Collaborate on treatment alterations based on the bits of knowledge inferred from computerized following apparatuses.

By grasping innovation, people with diabetes can change their self-management approach. These devices not as it were streamline following but too engage people to effectively lock in in their care, driving to more educated choices and moved forward generally well-being. Continuously counsel with healthcare professionals for direction on coordination innovation into your diabetes administration arrange.

Chapter 5 (Week 5)
Down to earth Dinner Arranging with The Diabetic Cookbook

Down to earth Dinner Arranging with "The Diabetic Cookbook" Supper arranging may be a vital viewpoint of overseeing diabetes, centering on adjusted nourishment to control blood sugar levels. "The Diabetic Cookbook" offers a riches of formulas planned for diabetes-friendly dinners. Here's a down to earth direct for dinner arranging utilizing this cookbook:

1. Build up Dietary Objectives:

• Recognize particular dietary objectives, such as accomplishing adjusted macronutrients, controlling parcel sizes, and consolidating an assortment of nutrient-dense nourishments.

2. Counsel with Healthcare Suppliers:

• Sometime recently beginning any unused feast arrange, counsel with healthcare suppliers to guarantee it adjusts with person wellbeing needs and dietary limitations.

3. Investigate Formula Alternatives:

• Browse "The Diabetic Cookbook" for formulas that coordinate dietary inclinations, counting primary dishes, sides, snacks, and pastries.

• Pay consideration to the dietary data given with each formula.

4. Center on Entirety Nourishments:

• Emphasize entire, natural nourishments wealthy in fiber, vitamins, and minerals.

• Consolidate incline proteins, vegetables, entirety grains, and sound fats into dinners.

5. Screen Carbohydrate Admissions:

• Be careful of carbohydrate admissions and select complex carbohydrates with a lower glycemic file.

• Utilize the cookbook's formulas that provide carbohydrate counts to disentangle dinner arranging.

6. Parcel Control:

• Hone parcel control to oversee calorie admissions and keep up a solid weight.

• Alter parcel sizes based on person vitality needs and blood sugar reactions.

7. Make Adjusted Suppers:

• Point for adjusted suppers that incorporate a combination of protein, solid fats, and carbohydrates.

• Utilize the cookbook's formulas that give a well-rounded wholesome profile.

8. Arrange Ahead:

• Arrange dinners for the week in development, considering variables like work plan, social occasions, and physical action.

• Planning in development can offer assistance guarantee adherence to the supper arrangement.

9. Expand Your Plate:

• Make different and colorful plates with an assortment of vegetables, proteins, and entire grains.

• Try with diverse flavors and cooking strategies.

10. Control Sodium and Sugar:

- Pay consideration to sodium and included sugar substance in formulas. - Select formulas that consolidate herbs, flavors, and characteristic flavors for taste.

11. Join Snacks:

Arrange for solid snacks between suppers to preserve steady blood sugar levels. - Investigate nibble formulas from the cookbook that adjust with dietary objectives.

12. Hydration:

- Prioritize hydration with water and other low-calorie refreshments. - Constrain the utilization of sugary drinks.

13. Customary Observing:

Frequently screen blood sugar levels to evaluate the effect of dinners on glycemic control. - Utilize the cookbook's formulas as an establishment for building dinners that back steady blood sugar.

14. Adjust Formulas to Inclinations:

Adjust formulas based on individual inclinations and dietary necessities. - Adjust ingredients or parcel sizes whereas guaranteeing dietary adjust.

15. Continuous Changes:

Execute continuous changes to permit for adjustment and supportability. - Try with unused formulas and steadily join them into the dinner arrange.

16. Look for Bolster:

Share feast plans and objectives with family or bolster systems. - Energize shared suppers that adjust with the diabetes-friendly standards of "The Diabetic Cookbook".

17. Customary Audit and Alteration:

Routinely survey the dinner plan's viability in accomplishing dietary objectives and blood sugar control. - Alter the arrangement as required, considering input from healthcare suppliers. Practical meal planning with "The Diabetic Cookbook" includes an adjusted and personalized approach. By joining an assortment of scrumptious and diabetes-friendly formulas, people can appreciate fulfilling dinners whereas successfully overseeing their blood sugar levels. Continuously counsel with healthcare experts for personalized exhortation and alterations based on person wellbeing contemplations.

The Significance of Feast Arranging in Diabetes Administration

Dinner arranging could be an essential component of successful diabetes administration, advertising an organized approach to nourishment that makes a difference direct blood sugar levels and advance generally well-being. Here are key reasons highlighting the significance of dinner arranging for people with diabetes:

1. Blood Sugar Control:

• Adjusting Supplements:

Feast arranging permits for the cautious determination and adjusting of carbohydrates, proteins, and fats, advancing steady blood sugar levels all through the day.

• Reliable Timing:

Standard and arranged suppers offer assistance keep up steady supplement admissions, decreasing the probability of extraordinary blood sugar changes.

2. Weight Administration:

• Parcel Control:

Dinner arranging empowers parcel control, supporting weight administration endeavors.

• Nutrient-Dense Choices:

Center on nutrient-dense nourishments makes a difference people keep up a healthy weight and prevent obesity-related complications.

3. Anticipation of Hypoglycemia and Hyperglycemia:

• Maintaining a strategic distance from Spikes:

Arranged suppers with controlled carbohydrate admissions offer assistance avoid post-meal hyperglycemia (tall blood sugar).

• Standard Snacking:

Joining arranged snacks makes a difference anticipate hypoglycemia (moo blood sugar) between dinners.

4. Personalized Sustenance:

• Custom fitted Approach:

Dinner arranging permits for the creation of personalized sustenance plans based on person dietary inclinations, social contemplations, and wellbeing needs.

• Obliging Inclinations:

People can adjust formulas and supper alternatives to suit their taste inclinations, making adherence to the arrangement more economical.

5. Controlled Admissions of Sugars and Prepared Nourishments:

• Minimizing Included Sugars:

Dinner arranging encourages the diminishment of included sugars and prepared nourishments, which can contribute to destitute blood sugar control.

• Choosing Entirety Nourishments:

Accentuation on entire, natural nourishments gives basic supplements without the negative affect of intemperate sugars.

6. Reliable Supplement Admissions:

• Supplement Assortment:

Arranging suppers guarantees an assortment of supplements, supporting generally wellbeing and anticipating supplement lacks.

• Reliable Caloric Admissions:

Regular meals and snacks maintain steady caloric admissions, anticipating vitality awkward nature.

7. Stretch Diminishment:

• Disposing of Choice Weakness:

Having a feast arrange kills the day by day push of choosing what to eat, making it less demanding to follow to dietary proposals.

• Productivity:

Planning dinners in development diminishes the time and exertion went through on every day food-related choices.

8. Budget-Friendly Choices:

• Smart Shopping:

Feast arranging includes making shopping records based on arranged dinners, advancing cost-effective and productive basic supply shopping.

• Minimizing Nourishment Squander:

Arranging makes a difference minimize nourishment squander by acquiring as it were the fundamental ingredients.

9. Instruction and Strengthening:

• Learning Wholesome Standards:

Dinner arranging includes learning around dietary standards and understanding the effect of diverse nourishments on blood sugar levels.

• Enabling People:

People ended up dynamic members in their care, picking up certainty in overseeing their condition through educated nourishment choices.

10. Long-Term Wellbeing Administration:

- Anticipating Complications:

Reliable blood sugar control through feast arranging contributes to the avoidance of long-term complications related with diabetes.

All-encompassing Wellbeing:

Meal planning is an all-encompassing approach to wellbeing administration, joining sustenance, physical movement, and way of life choices.

11. Bolster for Physical Action:

Optimizing Execution:

Well-planned suppers give the fundamental vitality and supplements to bolster physical action, contributing to by and large wellbeing and wellness.

Overseeing Blood Sugar Amid Work out:

Supper arranging makes a difference people make alterations to nourishment admissions some time recently, amid, and after work out for optimal blood sugar administration.

12. Collaborative Healthcare Approach:

Educated Healthcare Talks:

Feast arranging information can be shared with healthcare suppliers amid arrangements, cultivating educated discourses around dietary choices and alterations to treatment plans.

Therefore, supper arranging plays a significant part in diabetes administration by advancing blood sugar control, supporting weight administration, and contributing to in general well-being. People with diabetes, in collaboration with healthcare suppliers, can create personalized feast plans that adjust with their wellbeing objectives and inclinations. Normal observing, alterations, and continuous instruction contribute to the long-term victory of dinner arranging in diabetes care.

Making Adjusted Dinners

Making Adjusted Dinners for Diabetes Administration

Adjusted dinners are fundamental for people with diabetes to preserve stable blood sugar levels and bolster in general wellbeing. Here's a guide on how to make well-rounded and diabetes-friendly dinners:

1. Prioritize Entire, Natural Nourishments:

m• Select entirety grains, lean proteins, natural products, vegetables, and sound fats.

• Pick negligibly prepared alternatives to maximize supplement substance.

2. Take after the Plate Method:

• Isolate your plate into segments:

Half for non-starchy vegetables, a quarter for incline protein, and a quarter for entire grains or boring vegetables.

• This strategy makes a difference control parcel sizes and guarantees an adjusted blend of supplements.

3. Emphasize Non-Starchy Vegetables:

• Incorporate an assortment of colorful non-starchy vegetables such as verdant greens, broccoli, chime peppers, and cauliflower.

• These vegetables are wealthy in fiber, vitamins, and minerals without causing noteworthy spikes in blood sugar.

4. Incorporate Incline Proteins:

• Select incline protein sources like skinless poultry, angle, tofu, vegetables, and low-fat dairy items.

• Protein makes a difference with satiety and muscle support.

5. Decide on Solid Fats:

• Join sources of sound fats, such as avocados, nuts, seeds, and olive oil.

• These fats contribute to heart wellbeing and add flavor to dinners.

6. Control Carbohydrate Admissions:

• Center on complex carbohydrates with a moo glycemic file, such as entire grains, sweet potatoes, and vegetables.

• Screen parcel sizes to oversee carbohydrate admissions and avoid blood sugar spikes.

7. Be Careful of Parcel Sizes:

• Practice portion control to maintain a strategic distance from gorging.

• Utilize measuring instruments or visual prompts to appraise suitable parcel sizes.

8. Incorporate Fiber-Rich Nourishments:

• Select nourishments tall in dissolvable fiber, such as oats, beans, lentils, and natural products.

• Fiber makes a difference stabilize blood sugar levels and advances stomach related wellbeing.

9. Constrain Included Sugars and Handled Nourishments:

• Minimize the utilization of nourishments and refreshments with added sugars.

• Select entirety, characteristic sources of sweetness like natural products.

10. Screen Sodium Admissions:

Be careful of sodium substance, particularly in prepared and bundled nourishments. - Utilize herbs and flavors to flavor meals rather than over the top salt.

11. Remain Hydrated:

Drink plenty of water throughout the day. - Limit sugary drinks and pick for water, home grown tea, or imbued water.

12. Incorporate an Assortment of Nourishments:

Pivot nourishment choices to guarantee an assorted extend of supplements. - Explore with distinctive vegetables, proteins, and grains to keep dinners curiously.

13. Consider Dinner Timing:

Space dinners evenly throughout the day to assist control blood sugar levels.

Incorporate arranged snacks to anticipate long crevices between suppers.

14. Screen Blood Sugar Reactions:

Pay consideration to how diverse nourishments influence your blood sugar.

Standard observing makes a difference recognize designs and make educated alterations.

15. Customize to Person Needs:

Consider person inclinations, social impacts, and dietary confinements when arranging suppers.

Personalize formulas to suit taste inclinations and wellbeing objectives.

16. Plan Ahead:

Arrange suppers in progress to maintain a strategic distance from last-minute, less sound choices.

Plan and parcel dinners for simple get to amid active times.

17. Look for Proficient Direction:

Counsel with an enrolled dietitian or healthcare supplier for personalized meal planning advice. - Experts can give custom-made proposals based on person wellbeing needs.

18. Be Flexible and Appreciate Moderation:

Embrace flexibility in your feast arrange to suit different situations. - Permit for intermittent treats in balance to preserve an adjusted and maintainable approach to eating.

Creating balanced dinners could be a foundation of diabetes administration. By joining an assortment of nutrient-dense foods in fitting parcels, people with diabetes can accomplish ideal blood sugar control and bolster their by and large well-being. Continuously counsel with healthcare experts for personalized direction based on person wellbeing contemplations.

The Noteworthiness of Standard Eating Times in Diabetes Administration

Building up and maintaining normal eating times is pivotal for people with diabetes because it plays a critical part in overseeing blood sugar levels and generally wellbeing. Here are key reasons highlighting the significance of standard eating times:

1. Blood Sugar Direction:

• Reliable Supplement Admissions:

Standard eating times offer assistance convey supplement admissions equitably all through the day, avoiding huge variances in blood sugar levels.

• Avoiding Hypoglycemia:

Planned suppers and snacks offer assistance anticipate hypoglycemia (moo blood sugar) by dodging delayed periods without food.

2. Progressed Affront Affectability:

• Unfaltering Affront Discharge:

Eating at customary interims advances consistent affront discharge from the pancreas, improving the body's capacity to utilize glucose proficiently.

• Diminishing Affront Resistance:

Reliable dinner timing can contribute to diminishing affront resistance over time.

3. Overseeing Postprandial Blood Sugar:

• Controlled Spikes:

Normal dinners spread all through the day offer assistance control postprandial blood sugar spikes after eating.

• Adjusting Carbohydrates:

Disseminating carbohydrate admissions equitably underpins way better carbohydrate digestion system.

4. Supported Vitality Levels:

• Avoiding Vitality Lows:

Planned dinners and snacks offer assistance keep up steady vitality levels all through the day, anticipating weakness and vitality crashes.

• Optimizing Execution:

Relentless vitality underpins physical movement and in general well-being.

5. Craving Direction:

• Anticipating Indulging:

Customary suppers anticipate delayed periods of starvation, decreasing the probability of gorging amid consequent suppers.

• Adjusting Starvation Hormones:

Reliable eating times offer assistance control starvation hormones, advancing a more adjusted craving.

6. Weight Administration:

• Anticipating Motivation Eating:

Normal dinners diminish the probability of imprudent, undesirable nourishment choices.

• Supporting Parcel Control:

Organized eating times contribute to superior parcel control, supporting weight administration endeavors.

7. Metabolic Cadence:

• Circadian Rhythms:

The body's digestion system takes after circadian rhythms, and normal eating times adjust with these common cycles.

• Made strides Metabolic Productivity:

Eating in adjust with the body's inner clock can upgrade metabolic proficiency.

8. Superior Stomach related Wellbeing:

• Optimized Assimilation:

Normal eating times contribute to a more unsurprising stomach related cadence, advancing ideal supplement retention.

• Lessening Gastrointestinal Trouble:

Dividing suppers equitably makes a difference diminish the chance of heartburn and other gastrointestinal issues.

9. Mental Well-Being:

• Decreasing Stretch:

Unsurprising feast times diminish push related with sporadic eating designs or skipped dinners.

• Improving Schedule:

An organized eating schedule gives a sense of consistency and control.

10. Reliable Pharmaceutical Timing:

Synchronized with Medicines:

For people taking medicines or affront, customary eating times permit for way better synchronization with pharmaceutical plans. - Ideal Medicine Viability:

Steady supper timing bolsters the viability of diabetes medicines.

11. Building up Solid Propensities:

Making Schedule:

Customary eating times contribute to the foundation of solid eating propensities and schedules. - Long-Term Adherence:

Building up consistency cultivates long-term adherence to a sound eating arrange.

12. Supporting Rest Quality:

Adjusting Evening Snacks:

Arranging evening snacks at steady times can bolster way better blood sugar control amid the night, contributing to move forward rest quality.

13. Social and Social Viewpoints:

Improving Social Intuitive:

Organized eating times encourage social intelligent around suppers. - Adjusting with Social Hones:

Customary eating times can adjust with social standards and hones.

In view of the above, normal eating times are necessarily to diabetes administration, advancing steady blood sugar levels, supporting affront affectability, and contributing to generally well-being. Building up a steady eating schedule custom fitted to person inclinations and way of life may be a key component of a fruitful diabetes care arrange. Continuously counsel with healthcare experts for personalized direction based on person wellbeing contemplations.

The Diabetic Cookbook

Test Formulas

Certainly! Here are two test formulas from "The Diabetic Cookbook," outlined to be diabetes-friendly, nutritious, and tasty:

Formula 1:

Barbecued Lemon Herb Chicken with Simmered Vegetables

Ingredients:

• 4 boneless, skinless chicken breasts

• 2 tablespoons olive oil

• 1 lemon (zested and juiced)

• 2 teaspoons dried oregano

• 1 teaspoon dried thyme

• Salt and pepper to taste

For Broiled Vegetables:

• 1 zucchini, cut

• 1 ruddy chime pepper, cut

• 1 yellow chime pepper, cut

• 1 ruddy onion, cut

• 2 tablespoons olive oil

• Salt and pepper to taste

Instruction:

1. Preheat the barbecue to medium-high warm.

2. In a bowl, blend together olive oil, lemon pizzazz, lemon juice, oregano, thyme, salt, and pepper to form the marinade.

3. Put chicken breasts in a shallow dish and coat them with the marinade. Let it marinate for at slightest 30 minutes.

4. Whereas the chicken is marinating, preheat the stove to 400°F (200°C) for the broiled vegetables.

5. In an isolated bowl, hurl the cut zucchini, ruddy chime pepper, yellow chime pepper, and ruddy onion with olive oil, salt, and pepper.

6. Spread the vegetables on a heating sheet and cook for 20-25 minutes or until they are delicate and somewhat caramelized.

7. Barbecue the marinated chicken breasts for around 6-8 minutes per side or until completely cooked.

8. Serve the barbecued lemon herb chicken over a bed of the broiled vegetables.

Formula 2:

Quinoa and Dark Bean Serving of mixed greens

Ingredients:

• 1 glass quinoa, washed

• 2 mugs water

• 1 can (15 oz) dark beans, depleted and washed

• 1 glass cherry tomatoes, divided

• 1 cucumber, diced

• 1 ruddy onion, finely chopped

- 1/4 glass new cilantro, chopped

For the Dressing:

- 3 tablespoons olive oil

- 2 tablespoons lime juice

- 1 teaspoon ground cumin

- Salt and pepper to taste

Instructions:

1. In a medium pot, combine quinoa and water. Bring to a bubble, at that point diminish warm, cover, and stew for 15 minutes or until quinoa is cooked and water is ingested. Cushion with a fork and let it cool.

2. In an expansive bowl, combine the cooked quinoa, dark beans, cherry tomatoes, cucumber, ruddy onion, and cilantro.

3. In a little bowl, whisk together the olive oil, lime juice, ground cumin, salt, and pepper to make the dressing.

4. Pour the dressing over the quinoa blend and hurl until well combined.

5. Refrigerate the serving of mixed greens for at slightest 30 minutes some time recently serving to permit the flavors to merge.

6. Serve chilled as a reviving and nutritious side dish or light dinner.

These formulas exhibit the assortment and flavor that can be delighted in whereas keeping up a diabetes-friendly count calories. Continuously counsel with healthcare experts for personalized counsel based on person wellbeing contemplations.

Breakfast, Lunch, Supper, and Nibble Thoughts

Breakfast:

1. Greek Yogurt Parfait:

• Greek yogurt with berries (blueberries, strawberries).

• Sprinkle with a handful of almonds or walnuts.

• Sprinkle with a teaspoon of nectar.

2. Vegetable Omelet:

• Whisk together eggs and pour into a container.

• Include diced chime peppers, onions, spinach, and cherry tomatoes.

• Crease and cook until eggs are set.

3. Overnight Oats:

• Combine rolled oats with unsweetened almond drain.

• Include chia seeds, cut banana, and a touch of cinnamon.

• Refrigerate overnight and best with a couple of berries in the morning.

4. Entirety Grain Toast with Avocado:

• Toast a cut of whole-grain bread.

• Spread pounded avocado on beat.

• Sprinkle with a squeeze of salt and pepper.

Lunch:

1. Barbecued Chicken Serving of mixed greens:

• Flame broiled chicken breast over a bed of blended greens.

• Include cherry tomatoes, cucumber, and chime peppers.

• Dress with olive oil and balsamic vinegar.

2. Quinoa and Vegetable Bowl:

• Cooked quinoa with broiled vegetables (zucchini, chime peppers, cherry tomatoes).

• Beat with barbecued shrimp or tofu.

• Sprinkle with a lemon-tahini dressing.

3. Salmon Wrap:

• Barbecued or heated salmon with entire wheat or lettuce wraps.

• Include avocado, destroyed cabbage, and a crush of lime.

4. Turkey and Veggie Stir-Fry:

• Stir-fry incline ground turkey with broccoli, snap peas, and carrots.

• Season with low-sodium soy sauce and ginger.

• Serve over cauliflower rice.

Supper:

1. Prepared Cod with Asparagus:

• Season cod filets with lemon, garlic, and herbs.

• Prepare alongside asparagus lances until cooked through.

2. Veggie lover Chili:

• Blend dark beans, kidney beans, diced tomatoes, onions, and chime peppers.

• Include chili powder, cumin, and garlic.

• Stew until flavors merge.

3. Flame broiled Vegetable Sticks with Chicken:

• String chime peppers, cherry tomatoes, and chicken onto sticks.

• Flame broil until chicken is cooked and veggies are delicate.

4. Eggplant and Chickpea Curry:

• Sauté eggplant, chickpeas, and tomatoes in a curry sauce.

• Serve over cauliflower rice.

Snacks:

1. Apple Slices with Almond Butter:

• Cut apples and plunge in almond butter.

• A fulfilling combination of fiber and sound fats.

2. Vegetable Sticks with Hummus:

• Appreciate carrot, cucumber, and chime pepper sticks with hummus.

3. Hard-Boiled Eggs:

• A speedy and protein-rich nibble.

4. Nuts and Seeds Blend:

• Make a blend of almonds, walnuts, and pumpkin seeds.

Keep in mind to consider parcel sizes and screen blood sugar levels when attempting new foods. Adjust these ideas based on person inclinations and dietary prerequisites. Continuously counsel with healthcare experts for personalized counsel

Tips for Adjusting Favorite Formulas

Adjusting favorite formulas to create them diabetes-friendly includes making keen fixing choices and altering planning strategies. Here are a few tips for adjusting your favorite formulas:

1. Select Entirety Grains:

• Supplant refined grains with entire grains. Utilize brown rice, quinoa, entire wheat pasta, or entirety grain flour for a fiber-rich elective.

2. Alter Flour Types:

• Decide on almond flour, coconut flour, or oat flour rather than conventional all-purpose flour to lower the carbohydrate substance.

3. Diminish Included Sugars:

• Cut down on sugar by utilizing characteristic sweeteners like stevia, erythritol, or minister natural product.

• Increment sweetness with flavors like cinnamon or vanilla extricate.

4. Utilize Incline Proteins:

• Select incline cuts of meat and poultry.

• Consolidate plant-based protein sources like tofu, tempeh, or vegetables.

5. Solid Fats:

• Substitute immersed fats with more beneficial alternatives like olive oil, avocado oil, or nut oils.

• Include sources of omega-3 fatty acids, such as greasy angle or flaxseeds.

6. Parcel Control:

• Be careful of parcel sizes to oversee carbohydrate admissions.

• Use smaller plates to assist control generally parcels.

7. Increment Fiber:

• Include more fiber to your formulas with vegetables, vegetables, and entirety grains.

• Consider including flaxseeds or chia seeds to boost fiber substance.

8. Select Low-Glycemic Ingredients:

• Select low-glycemic record nourishments to assist manage blood sugar levels.

• For case, choose sweet potatoes over standard potatoes.

9. Alter Cooking Strategies:

• Flame broil, heat, steam, or roast rather than searing to diminish included fats.

• Utilize non-stick cooking shower or little sums of solid oils.

10. Sodium Awareness:

• Constrain salt admissions by utilizing

herbs, flavors, and other flavorings.

• Select low-sodium or no-salt-added forms of ingredients.

11. Dairy Choices:

• Prefer low-fat or fat-free dairy items.

• Investigate non-dairy options like almond drain or coconut drain.

12. Careful Dessert Choices:

• Explore with sugar-free or low-sugar dessert recipes.

• Consider utilizing natural product as a common sweetener in sweets.

13. Try with Substitutes:

• Investigate fixing substitutes, such as cauliflower rice instead of standard rice or zucchini noodles rather than pasta.

• Use squashed cauliflower rather than pounded potatoes.

14. Studied Sustenance Names:

• Check nutritional data on bundled ingredients.

• Explore for lower-carb and lower-sugar alternatives.

15. Customize Formulas:

• Do not be perplexed to make alterations based on your taste inclinations and dietary needs.

• Explore with different flavors and flavors to enhance the taste of your dishes.

16. Test and Alter:

• When adjusting a formula, test the altered adaptation and alter as required.

• Keep a record of fruitful adjustments for future utilize.

17. Counsel with a Dietitian:

• Seek guidance from an enlisted dietitian or healthcare proficient for personalized counsel on adjusting formulas.

Keep in mind to screen your blood sugar levels after attempting unused formulas and adjustments to get it how they influence your body. Making slow changes and joining assortment into your slim down can contribute to a feasible and enjoyable eating arrange. Continuously counsel with healthcare experts for personalized counsel based on person wellbeing contemplations

Chapter 6 (Week 6)
Long-Term Procedures for Diabetes Administration

Long-term methodologies for diabetes administration include embracing an all-encompassing approach to preserve by and large wellbeing and anticipate complications. Here are key methodologies for compelling long-term diabetes administration:

1. Sound Eating:

• Take after an adjusted and nutritious count calories that centers on entire nourishments, counting natural products, vegetables, incline proteins, and entirety grains.

• Control parcel sizes and screen carbohydrate admissions.

• Select nourishments with a low glycemic list to assist oversee blood sugar levels.

2. Normal Physical Movement:

• Lock in in standard physical movement, counting oxygen consuming works out (strolling, swimming, cycling) and quality preparing.

• Point for at slightest 150 minutes of moderate-intensity work out per week.

• Counsel with healthcare experts some time recently beginning a modern workout regimen.

3. Weight Administration:

• Keep up a solid weight through a combination of an adjusted count calories and normal work out.

• Set practical weight misfortune objectives on the off chance that required, as indeed unassuming weight misfortune can have critical benefits for blood sugar control.

4. Normal Blood Sugar Checking:

• Screen blood sugar levels frequently, as exhorted by healthcare experts.

• Keep track of designs and variances to form educated choices approximately diet, exercise, and pharmaceutical alterations.

5. Pharmaceutical Adherence:

• Take endorsed drugs as coordinated by healthcare suppliers.

• Communicate any concerns or side impacts with healthcare experts.

• Take after up routinely to survey pharmaceutical adequacy and potential alterations.

6. Push Administration:

• Hone stress-reducing strategies, such as profound breathing, contemplation, yoga, or mindfulness.

• Oversee stretch to avoid potential impacts on blood sugar levels.

7. Standard Restorative Check-Ups:

• Plan customary check-ups with healthcare suppliers to screen in general wellbeing.

• Address any concerns or changes in wellbeing instantly.

8. Foot Care:

• Review feet day by day for any signs of harm, contamination, or changes.

• Keep feet clean and moisturized.

• Wear comfortable, well-fitting shoes and check for legitimate circulation.

9. Eye Care:

• Go to standard eye exams to distinguish and address any diabetic eye complications.

• Report any changes in vision or eye wellbeing expeditiously.

10. Dental Wellbeing:

• Keep up great verbal cleanliness to avoid dental issues related with diabetes.

• Plan customary dental check-ups.

11. Rest Cleanliness:

• Prioritize good sleep propensities to back in general wellbeing.

• Point for 7-9 hours of quality rest each night.

12. Instruction and Bolster:

• Remain educated approximately diabetes administration through instruction programs and assets.

• Look for back from healthcare experts, diabetes teachers, and bolster bunches.

13. Standard Inoculations:

• Remain up-to-date on immunizations, including flu shots and other immunizations prescribed for people with diabetes.

14. Way of life Alterations:

• Stopped smoking in the event that pertinent, as smoking can worsen diabetes-related complications.

• Restrain liquor utilization and make educated choices around its effect on blood sugar levels.

15. Individualized Care Arrange:

• Work with healthcare experts to create an individualized diabetes care arrange that considers individual wellbeing objectives, inclinations, and way of life.

16. Mindfulness of Mental Wellbeing:

• Be careful of mental wellbeing and look for bolster for enthusiastic well-being.

• Address any signs of discouragement or uneasiness expeditiously.

17. Community Engagement:

• Interface with diabetes bolster bunches and communities to share encounters and experiences.

• Construct a strong organize of companions and family.

Long-term diabetes administration may be a long lasting commitment that includes reliable self-care hones and collaboration with healthcare experts. Personalized care plans, normal checking, and a center on in general well-being contribute to fruitful long-term administration and distant better; a much better; a higher; a stronger; an improved quality of life. Continuously counsel with healthcare professionals for personalized exhortation based on person wellbeing contemplations.

Building up a Schedule

Setting up a schedule is significant for successful diabetes administration. A steady daily routine makes a difference control blood sugar levels, bolsters medicine adherence, and advances in general well-being. Here's a direct to assist set up a schedule:

1. Set Standard Supper Times:

• Arrange breakfast, lunch, supper, and snacks at reliable times each day.

• Point for equitably dispersed suppers to assist oversee blood sugar levels.

2. Adjust Supplements:

• Incorporate a blend of carbohydrates, proteins, and sound fats in each feast.

• Select entirety, natural nourishments for adjusted nourishment.

3. Remain Hydrated:

• Drink bounty of water all through the day.

• Constrain sugary refreshments and choose water, home grown tea, or infused water.

4. Customary Physical Movement:

• Schedule regular work out sessions.

• Incorporate a blend of oxygen consuming works out, quality preparing, and adaptability works out.

5. Blood Sugar Observing:

• Set up a schedule for checking blood sugar levels.

• Consistency in monitoring makes a difference distinguish designs and make opportune alterations.

6. Pharmaceutical Adherence:

• Take medicines at the same time each day.

• Use pill organizers or medicine updates to remain on track.

7. Dinner Arranging and Prep:

• Arrange suppers for the week and plan ingredients in development.

• Bunch cooking can spare time and guarantee get to to solid choices.

8. Prioritize Rest:

• Point for 7-9 hours of quality rest each night.

• Establish a sleep time schedule to advance superior rest.

9. Stretch Administration:

• Consolidate stress-reducing exercises such as profound breathing, contemplation, or mindfulness.

• Plan customary breaks to unwind and energize.

10. Foot and Skin Care:

11. Normal Restorative Check-Ups: arrangements with healthcare experts. - Keep track of check-up dates and screenings.

12. Dental Wellbeing suggested.

13. Eye Care:

14. Record Keeping:

15. Adaptability:

16. Bolster Framework:

17. Standard Survey:

18. Teach Yourself:

19. Celebrate Little Wins:

20. Look for Proficient Direction:

Establishing and keeping up a schedule requires commitment and flexibility. A well-structured schedule contributes to way better blood sugar control, progressed in general wellbeing, and improved quality of life. Continuously counsel with healthcare experts for personalized exhortation based on person wellbeing contemplations.

Making Day by day Diabetes Administration Propensities

Making day by day propensities for diabetes management includes consolidating reliable, health-promoting behaviors into your schedule. Here are basic day by day propensities to back viable diabetes administration:

1. Customary Blood Sugar Checking:

• Check blood sugar levels as suggested by your healthcare supplier.

• Utilize a blood glucose meter and keep a log to track designs.

2. Adjusted Supper Arranging:

• Arrange suppers that incorporate an adjustment of carbohydrates, proteins, and sound fats.

• Choose whole, natural nourishments and control parcel sizes.

3. Consistent Meal Times:

• Build up customary supper times and avoid skipping suppers.

• Space suppers equally all through the day to assist direct blood sugar levels.

4. Physical Movement:

• Consolidate customary work out into your schedule.

• Aim for a blend of high-impact works out, quality preparing, and adaptability works out.

5. Pharmaceutical Adherence:

• Take endorsed solutions at the same time each day.

• Utilize pill organizers or smartphone updates to remain on plan.

6. Hydration:

• Drink bounty of water all through the day.

• Limit sugary refreshments and elect water, home grown tea, or imbued water.

7. Nutrient-Dense Snacking:

• Select sound snacks like nuts, seeds, vegetables, or Greek yogurt.

• Be careful of parcel sizes and dodge high-sugar snacks.

8. Stretch Administration:

• Hone stress-reducing methods such as profound breathing, reflection, or mindfulness.

• Plan breaks amid the day to unwind and energize.

9. Foot Care:

• Review feet every day for any signs of damage, redness, or changes.

• Moisturize feet routinely and wear comfortable, well-fitting shoes.

10. Rest Cleanliness:

11. Standard Restorative Check-Ups:

12. Dental Health:

13. Eye Care:

14. Record Keeping:

- Keep a diabetes diary to track suppers, work out, solutions, and blood sugar levels. - Share records with healthcare providers amid arrangements.

15. Sound Cooking and Supper Prep:

- Cook nourishments.

16. Constrain Liquor Utilization:

17. Remain Informed: diabetes care.

18. Mental Wellbeing Mindfulness:

19. Blood Weight Administration:

20. Celebrate Victory:

Recognize and celebrate little triumphs in your diabetes administration travel. - Positive support cultivates long-term commitment.

Building up these day by day propensities cultivates a proactive and all-encompassing approach to diabetes administration. Consistency is key, and over time, these propensities can ended up a fundamentally portion of your way of, life contributing to superior wellbeing results. Continuously counsel with healthcare experts for personalized exhortation based on person health considerations.

Adjusting Diabetes Care with Standard Of living

Adjusting diabetes care with way of life is fundamental for keeping up in general well-being and effectively overseeing the condition. Here are commonsense tips to coordinated diabetes care seamlessly into your day by day schedule:

1. Consolidate Solid Suppers:

• Arrange suppers in development and make sound nourishment choices.

• Plan adjusted dinners that adjust with your dietary inclinations.

2. Convenient Snacks:

• Keep diabetes-friendly snacks on hand for helpful, healthy munching.

• Want choices like nuts, seeds, or cut-up vegetables.

3. Supper Timing:

• Build up normal dinner times and space them evenly throughout the day.

• Arrange suppers that adjust along with your everyday plan.

4. Physical Action Integration:

• Integrate physical action into your schedule.

• Select exercises you enjoy to form work out a portion of your way of life.

5. Medicine Adherence:

• Utilize pill organizers or smartphone reminders for consistent medicine adherence.

• Carry drugs with you for simple get to.

6. Hydration Mindfulness:

• Keep a water bottle with you all through the day.

• Restrain sugary drinks and prioritize water, home grown tea, or infused water.

7. Stress Administration Strategies:

• Practice push administration procedures, such as profound breathing or mindfulness.

• Recognize stress triggers and create techniques to address them.

8. Foot Care Propensities:

• Check your feet day by day for any signs of damage or changes.

• Make foot care part of your day by day cleanliness schedule.

9. Quality Rest:

• Prioritize great rest cleanliness to back in general wellbeing.

• Set up a calming bedtime schedule for way better rest quality.

10. Schedule Blood Sugar Checks:

- Set updates for schedule blood sugar checks. - Keep a blood glucose meter easily accessible.

11. Supper Prep for Comfort:

- Arrange and prep suppers in development to spare time amid active days. - Utilize batch cooking for proficient supper planning.

12. Standard Restorative Check-Ups:

13. Dental and Eye Care Integration:

- Plan dental and eye care arrangements ahead of time. - Make these arrangements portion of your schedule healthcare arrange.

14. Workplace Strategies:

- Communicate with colleagues about your diabetes management needs. - Keep snacks, solutions, and necessary supplies at your working environment.

15. Versatility:

- Be adaptable and adaptable to changes in your schedule. - Have contingency plans for unforeseen occasions.

16. Community and Family Inclusion:

- Share your diabetes administration arrange with family and companions. - Involve cherished ones in steady exercises like strolls or sound feast arranging.

17. Careful Choices:

- Be mindful of your choices throughout the day. - Make choices that adjust together with your diabetes care objectives.

18. Travel Arranging:

- Plan ahead for travel, guaranteeing you have sufficient medicines and supplies. - Familiarize yourself with nearby healthcare assets at your goal.

19. Positive Fortification:

- Celebrate accomplishments and milestones in your diabetes administration travel. - Positive fortification cultivates a positive outlook.

20. Instructive Progression:

- Remain educated almost diabetes administration through persistent instruction. - Go to workshops or programs to improve your knowledge.

Balancing diabetes care with way of life is almost making cognizant choices that prioritize wellbeing while allowing for flexibility and enjoyment in every day exercises. With consistent effort, these propensities can ended up moment nature, making a harmonious integration of diabetes care into your generally way of life. Continuously counsel with healthcare professionals for personalized exhortation based on person wellbeing contemplations.

Passionate Wellness

• Adapting with Stretch and Passionate Challenges

Adapting with push and enthusiastic challenges is vital for by and large well-being, particularly for people overseeing diabetes. Here are down to earth methodologies to assist explore stretch and enthusiastic challenges:

1. Mindfulness and Unwinding Procedures:

• Hone profound breathing works out, contemplation, or guided symbolism to advance unwinding.

• Lock in in mindfulness activities to remain show within the minute.

2. Normal Work out:

• Join normal physical movement into your schedule.

• Work out discharges endorphins, which can make strides disposition and decrease push.

3. Social Bolster:

• Interface with companions, family, or bolster bunches.

• Share your sentiments and concerns with somebody you believe.

4. Helpful Bolster:

• Consider talking to a specialist or counselor.

• Proficient back can give important adapting techniques.

5. Journaling:

• Keep a diary to specific your considerations and feelings.

• Reflecting on your sentiments can offer assistance handle and get it them.

6. Pastimes and Inventive Outlets:

• Lock in in exercises you appreciate, whether it's craftsmanship, music, or cultivating.

• Imaginative outlets can serve as a restorative discharge.

7. Setting up Boundaries:

• Set clear boundaries to oversee stressors.

• Learn to say no when vital and prioritize self-care.

8. Solid Way of life Choices:

• Keep up an adjusted slim down and remain hydrated.

• Guarantee you get sufficient rest to bolster enthusiastic well-being.

9. Time Administration:

• Prioritize errands and break them into sensible steps.

• Maintain a strategic distance from over-burdening your plan and apportion time for self-care.

10. Positive Confirmations: accomplishments.

11. Problem-Solving Abilities:

- Create compelling problem-solving abilities. - Break down challenges into littler, significant steps.

12. Cognitive Behavioral Methods:

- Learn and hone cognitive-behavioral procedures. - Challenge negative contemplations and supplant them with positive ones.

13. Acknowledgment and Commitment Treatment (ACT):

- Grasp acknowledgment and commit to positive activities. - Center on values and take steps adjusted with those values.

14. Time for Self-Reflection:

- Distribute time for self-reflection. - Get it your feelings and distinguish designs.

15. Otherworldly Hones:

- Lock in in otherworldly hones that bring consolation and peace. - This seem incorporate supplication, contemplation, or going to devout administrations.

16. Chuckling and Humor:

- Discover minutes of bliss and chuckling in daily life.
- Chuckling can be an effective push reliever.

17. Nature and Open air Exercises:

- Spend time in nature or lock in in open air exercises.
- New discuss and characteristic environment can have a calming impact.

18. Volunteer Work:

- Consider locks in in volunteer exercises. - Making a difference others can give a sense of reason and fulfillment.

19. Looking for Proficient Exhortation:

- On the off chance that required, counsel with a mental wellbeing proficient. - They can give specialized direction and back.

20. Mind-Body Practices:

- Investigate mind-body hones such as yoga or tai chi.
- These exercises advance unwinding and push lessening.

Adapting with push is an ongoing process, and finding what works best for you'll include attempting distinctive techniques. Prioritize self-care, be quiet with yourself, and look for bolster when required. Continuously counsel with healthcare and mental wellbeing experts for personalized exhortation based on person wellbeing contemplations

Looking for Extra Back

Looking for extra back may be a crucial step for people overseeing diabetes, particularly when confronting challenges that affect passionate well-being and by and large wellbeing. Here are various roads for looking for back:

1. Healthcare Professionals:

• Counsel along with your healthcare group, counting your essential care doctor, endocrinologist, or diabetes teacher.

• Examine any enthusiastic challenges or stressors influencing your diabetes administration.

2. Mental Wellbeing Experts:

• Look for the direction of mental wellbeing experts such as clinicians, counselors, or advisors.

• They can give custom fitted methodologies for overseeing stretch and enthusiastic challenges.

3. Diabetes Back Groups:

• Connect diabetes back bunches in your community or online.

• Interfacing with others confronting comparable challenges can offer understanding and shared encounters.

4. Family and Friends:

• Share your sentiments with trusted family individuals and companions.

• Their bolster can give enthusiastic consolation and support.

5. Online Communities:

• Take an interest in online gatherings and communities committed to diabetes administration.

• Lock in in talks, inquire questions, and learn from others' encounters.

6. Wellbeing and Wellness Programs:

• Investigate wellbeing and wellness programs that incorporate both physical and mental well-being.

• These programs may offer an all-encompassing approach to diabetes administration.

7. Devout or Otherworldly Pioneers:

• Seek direction from devout or otherworldly pioneers.

• Many communities have assets that address enthusiastic well-being and adapting.

8. Representative Help Programs (EAP):

• In the event that pertinent, utilize worker help programs given by your work environment.

• EAPs frequently offer counseling administrations and assets.

9. Apps and Innovation:

• Utilize apps and online stages planned to back mental wellbeing and well-being.

• A few apps center on stretch diminishment, reflection, or mindfulness.

10. Community Centers:

11. Instructive Workshops:

12. Hotlines and Helplines:

- Reach out to hotlines or helplines specializing in mental wellbeing bolster. - Experts are accessible to provide prompt help and direction.

13. Restorative Apps:

- Investigate helpful apps that offer guided reflection, unwinding works out, or cognitive-behavioral devices. - A few apps are particularly outlined for overseeing stretch and uneasiness.

14. Books and Writing:

- Read books and writing centered on passionate well-being and diabetes management. - Numerous creators share individual encounters and adapting procedures.

15. National Diabetes Organizations:

16. Patient Advocacy Bunches:

17. Online Courses: relevant courses.

18. Money related Counseling Administrations:

- In case monetary stressors affect your well-being, consider looking for monetary counseling administrations. - Numerous organizations give help in overseeing budgetary challenges.

19. Telehealth Administrations:

- Investigate telehealth administrations for virtual counseling or treatment sessions. - Telehealth permits for helpful get to to mental wellbeing experts.

20. Understanding Pilots:

- A few healthcare frameworks offer understanding pilots or facilitators. - These professionals can direct you to significant assets and bolster administrations.

Keep in mind, looking for back could be a sign of strength, and there are different resources available to help you. Select the choices that adjust along with your inclinations and needs, and do not delay to reach out when essential. Continuously counsel with healthcare and mental wellbeing professionals for personalized exhortation based on person wellbeing contemplations.

Conclusion
Reflection on the 6-Week Travel

Reflection on a 6-week travel of exploring type 1 diabetes and joining "The Diabetic Cookbook and Supper Arrange" involves considering the advance made, challenges confronted, and lessons learned. Here's an intelligent outline:

Advance and Accomplishments:

1. Progressed Blood Sugar Control:

• Reflect on any positive changes in blood sugar levels.

• Note occurrences of soundness and decreased changes.

2. Dietary Victories:

• Recognize fruitful adherence to an adjusted and diabetes-friendly count calories.

• Celebrate finding modern, delightful formulas and dinners.

3. Built up Schedule:

• Assess the adequacy of the set up schedule for meals, drugs, and work out.

• Note any advancements in schedule adherence.

4. Physical Activity Integration:

• Reflect on the integration of regular physical movement into the daily routine.

• Recognize any positive impacts on in general well-being.

5. Mindfulness and Stretch Administration:

• Assess the adequacy of push administration methods.

• Recognize minutes of mindfulness and their effects on passionate well-being.

6. Adherence to Pharmaceutical:

• Reflect on reliable adherence to endorsed solutions.

• Recognize any adjustments made in discussion with healthcare experts.

7. Instructive Development:

• Consider the information picked up approximately diabetes administration.

• Reflect on any educational materials or assets that were especially accommodating.

Challenges Faced

1. Dietary Alterations:

• Distinguish particular challenges experienced whereas adjusting to a modern dietary approach.

• Consider procedures for overcoming these challenges.

2. Enthusiastic and Mental Well-Being:

• Reflect on minutes of enthusiastic push or mental challenges.

• Investigate adapting instruments that were compelling or zones for enhancement.

3. Consistency in Schedule:

• Recognize any battles with keeping up a reliable schedule.

• Identify potential obstructions and brainstorm arrangements.

4. Physical Action Challenges:

• Consider any obstacles confronted in coordination customary work out.

• Investigate alterations or modifications to overcome challenges.

5. Exploring Social Circumstances:

• Reflect on encounters with social circumstances including nourishment.

• Consider procedures for overseeing these circumstances more viably.

6. Observing and Record Keeping:

• Assess the consistency of blood sugar observing and record-keeping.

• Identify any areas for change in following wellbeing measurements.

Lessons Learned

1. Personalized Approaches:

• Get it the significance of fitting diabetes administration to individual needs.

• Recognize that what works for one person may vary from others.

2. Persistent Learning:

• Grasp an attitude of persistent learning around diabetes administration.

• Appreciate the advancing nature of information within the field.

3. Adaptability and Versatility:

• Learn the esteem of being flexible and versatile within the confront of challenges.

• Get it that alterations may be fundamental based on changing circumstances.

4. Self-Advocacy:

• Recognize the significance of supporting for individual wellbeing needs.

• Understand the role of compelling communication with healthcare experts.

5. Bolster Systems:

• Recognize the significance of back frameworks, whether from companions, family, or healthcare suppliers.

• Get it the effect of a supportive community on generally well-being.

6. All-encompassing Well-Being:

• Realize the interconnecting of physical, enthusiastic, and mental well-being.

• Consider the all-encompassing approach to health in diabetes administration.

7. Celebrating Little Wins:

• Learn to celebrate little triumphs and achievements.

• Get it the positive affect of recognizing advance.

Moving Forward

1. Objective Setting:

• Reflect on long-term objectives for diabetes management.

• Consider setting achievable, practical objectives for proceeded advance.

2. Building on Victory:

• Recognize viewpoints of the travel that have been especially effective.

• Explore ways to construct on these victories for maintained advance.

3. Nonstop Bolster:

• Recognize the ongoing need for back from healthcare experts, back bunches, and cherished ones.

• Consider ways to preserve a solid bolster arrange.

4. Embracing Change:

• Grasp the thought that overseeing diabetes includes a nonstop process of adaptation.

• Get it that alterations and changes are a natural part of the travel.

5. Looking for Proficient Direction:

• Reaffirm the significance of looking for direction from healthcare professionals.

• Plan customary check-ups and meetings to guarantee proceeded bolster.

6. Keeping up Inspiration:

• Develop a positive attitude within the confront of challenges.

• Recognize that maintaining a positive viewpoint contributes to by and large well-being.

Reflection on the 6-week travel gives profitable bits of knowledge for future diabetes administration. It serves as an establishment for continued growth, adjustment, and an all-encompassing approach to overall health. Always counsel with healthcare experts for personalized exhortation based on person wellbeing contemplations.

Looking Ahead

Economical Hones for Long-Term Wellness

Looking ahead, maintainable hones for long-term wellness in overseeing type 1 diabetes include embracing propensities that contribute to generally wellbeing and well-being. Here are key contemplations and hones to cultivate maintainable wellness:

1. All-encompassing Approach:

• Embrace an all-encompassing approach that addresses physical, mental, and enthusiastic well-being.

• Get it the interconnecting of different perspectives of wellbeing.

2. Personalized Care:

• Proceed to tailor diabetes administration to person needs and preferences.

• Collaborate with healthcare professionals to make a personalized care arrange.

3. Nutrient-Rich Count calories:

• Maintain a nutrient-rich slim down that underpins in general wellbeing.

• Proceed investigating and joining assorted, diabetes-friendly formulas.

4. Reliable Physical Action:

• Integrate regular physical activity into existence.

• Select exercises that adjust with personal interface to guarantee long-term adherence.

5. Standard Checking:

• Support standard blood sugar checking and record-keeping.

• Utilize innovation and apps to streamline tracking forms.

6. Mindfulness Hones:

• Develop mindfulness hones for push administration.

• Join exercises such as contemplation or profound breathing into day by day schedules.

7. Passionate Well-Being:

• Prioritize enthusiastic well-being and look for bolster when required.

• Proceed locks in with back systems, counting companions, family, and healthcare experts.

8. Long lasting Learning:

• Keep up a commitment to ceaseless learning around diabetes administration.

• Remain educated approximately progressions, unused inquire about, and advancing best hones.

9. Customary Check-Ups:

• Plan normal check-ups with healthcare suppliers.

• Address any concerns expeditiously and proactively oversee wellbeing.

10. Adaptability and Versatility:

- Grasp adaptability and versatility in overseeing diabetes. - Get it that alterations to the care arrange may be fundamental over time.

11. Maintainable Schedules:

- Set up

12. Objective Setting:

13. Building Versatility: mentality and center on arrangements instead of deterrents.

14. Peer Back: others overseeing diabetes.

15. Rest Cleanliness:

16. Customary Work out Assortment: an assortment of works out to avoid repetitiveness. - Investigate unused exercises to keep physical movement pleasant.

17. Standard Dental and Eye Check-Ups:

18. Mind-Body Hones:

19. Positive Support:

- Hone positive support and celebrate victories. - Recognize endeavors and accomplishments in overseeing diabetes.

20. Long-Term Point of view:

21. Adjustment to Innovative Propels:

- Remain educated around innovative progressions in diabetes care. - Consider joining modern instruments and gadgets that improve administration.

22. Community Engagement:

- Lock in with the diabetes community and backing endeavors. - Contribute to raising mindfulness and supporting others.

23. Monetary Wellness:

- Consider monetary wellness as portion of by and large well-being. - Look for assets or help for overseeing healthcare costs.

24. Normal Inoculations:

- Remain up-to-date on inoculations and preventive healthcare measures. - Consult with healthcare experts around prescribed immunizations.

25. Positive Way of life Propensities:

- Develop positive way of life propensities that contribute to generally wellbeing. - Center on propensities that advance well-being past diabetes administration.

Feasible hones for long-term wellness include a commitment to self-care, persistent learning, and a versatile attitude. By joining these hones into existence, people with type 1 diabetes can cultivate flexibility and keep up ideal wellbeing over a long time. Continuously counsel with healthcare experts for personalized exhortation based on person wellbeing contemplations.

Glossary of Diabetes Terms

1. A1C (HbA1c):

A degree of normal blood glucose levels over the past two to three months, showing long-term blood sugar control.

2. Beta Cells:

Cells within the pancreas that create and discharge affront.

3. Blood Glucose:

The concentration of glucose (sugar) display within the blood, measured in milligrams per deciliter (mg/dL) or millimoles per liter (mmol/L).

4. Bolus:

A dosage of rapid-acting affront taken to cover the carbohydrates expended in a feast or to adjust tall blood sugar.

5. Carbohydrate (Carb):

A macronutrient found in nourishment that is broken down into glucose and utilized as a vitality source.

6. Persistent Glucose Monitoring (CGM):

A framework that persistently tracks blood glucose levels all through the day, giving real-time information.

7. Diabetes Mellitus:

An inveterate condition characterized by raised blood glucose levels due to the body's failure to create or successfully utilize affront.

8. Affront:

A hormone created by the pancreas that regulates blood sugar by encouraging the assimilation of glucose into cells.

9. Glucagon:

A hormone delivered by the pancreas that raises blood sugar levels by invigorating the discharge of glucose from the liver.

10. Gestational Diabetes:

Diabetes that creates amid pregnancy and can increment the chance of complications for both the mother and child.

11. Hyperglycemia:

Tall blood sugar levels, frequently characterized by side effects such as expanded thirst, visit urination, and weariness.

12. Hypoglycemia:

Moo blood sugar levels, driving to indications like shakiness, disarray, and peevishness.

13. Ketoacidosis:

A genuine condition where the body produces tall levels of ketones, ordinarily seen in uncontrolled diabetes.

14. Lancet:

A little, sharp instrument utilized to prick the skin for blood glucose testing.

15. Metformin:

A verbal medicine commonly endorsed to oversee blood sugar levels in individuals with type 2 diabetes.

16. Pancreas:

An organ that produces affront and other hormones included in absorption and blood sugar direction.

17. Prediabetes:

A condition where blood glucose levels are higher than typical but not tall sufficient to be analyzed as diabetes.

18. Type 1 Diabetes:

An immune system condition where the resistant framework assaults and crushes the insulin-producing beta cells within the pancreas.

19. Type 2 Diabetes:

A condition where the body's cells gotten to be safe to affront, and the pancreas can't create sufficient affront to compensate.

20. Microvascular Complications:

Diabetes-related complications influencing little blood vessels, counting retinopathy (eye harm) and nephropathy (kidney harm).

21. Macrovascular Complications:

Diabetes-related complications influencing huge blood vessels, expanding the chance of heart illness and stroke.

22. Neuropathy:

Nerve harm, a common complication of diabetes that can lead to shivering, torment, and deadness, frequently within the limits.

23. Hypertension:

Tall blood weight, a common comorbidity in people with diabetes.

24. Polyphagia:

Intemperate starvation, an indication regularly related with tall blood sugar levels.

25. Polydipsia:

Over the top thirst, an indication regularly related with tall blood sugar levels.